The New Medicine and the Old Ethics

The
New Medicine
and the
Old Ethics

ALBERT R. JONSEN

Harvard University Press
Cambridge, Massachusetts
London, England
1990

This book is printed on acid-free paper, and its binding materials have been chosen for strength and durability.

LIBRARY OF CONGRESS CATALOGING-IN-PUBLICATION DATA
Jonsen, Albert R.
    The new medicine and the old ethics / Albert R. Jonsen. p.   cm.
    Includes bibliographical references (p.   ).
    ISBN 0-674-61725-8 (alk. paper)
    1. Medical ethics. I. Title.
R724.J663   1990
174'.2—dc20   90-33157
                        CIP

For my uncle, Charles F. Sweigert,

*who during forty-seven years of medical practice (1930–1977)
watched the new medicine meet the old ethics—a physician who,
in the words of Sir William Osler, combined "a stern sense of duty
with the mental freshness of youth"*

Preface

The new medicine has hard, sharp edges: its instruments, machines, and drugs have a technological precision that makes possible remarkably accurate diagnosis and therapy. We have learned, however, that the precision and the accuracy raise many ethical questions. Unlike the hard edges of the new medicine, the ethical questions have a blurred outline. Our discussions of responsibility, rights, duties, interests, beneficence, and justice may be eloquent, even fervent, but are rarely conclusive. Ever since René Descartes championed "the clear and distinct idea" as the ideal of philosophical reasoning, philosophers have endeavored to hone the meanings of these ethical terms. One of Descartes's eminent early disciples, Baruch Spinoza, was a lens grinder; he wanted moral truths to sparkle like his cut glass and to have the precision of the geometric axioms that informed his optics. He even wrote a book entitled *Ethics Proven by the Method of Geometry*.

After several centuries of philosophical lens grinding and concept sharpening, we are still beset by cloudy blurs and soft edges around ethical ideas. Our incessant arguments bear witness to the failure of the geometric method in morality. But this failure need not push us into skepticism. It can remind us that before Descartes and Spinoza, many renowned thinkers were tolerant of blurred edges. Greatest among them was Aristotle, who commenced his *Nicomachean Ethics* with this caution:

> Our discussion will be adequate if it achieves clarity within the limits of the subject matter. For precision cannot be expected in the treatment of all subjects alike, any more than it can be expected in all manufactured articles. Problems of what is noble and just . . . present much variety and irregularity . . . so that the well-educated man is one who searches for that degree of precision in each kind of study which the nature of the subject admits: it is just as foolish to accept arguments of probability from a mathematician as to demand strict demonstrations from an orator. (I.3.1094b)

Aristotle was a physician's son. Perhaps, as a perceptive child, he noticed his father puzzling through the diagnosis of a patient's illness and cautiously selecting one of many treatment options. Years later, when he wrote about ethics, the comparison with medicine came to his mind:

> Matters of practical conduct have nothing invariable about them, any more than matters of health. This is true of ethics in general, and it is true even more of moral issues arising in particular cases. These are not a scientific or technical matter: rather as in medicine or navigation, they require human beings to consider what is appropriate to specific circumstances and to specific occasions. (II.2.1104a)

Mine is a book that inclines to Aristotle rather than Descartes and Spinoza. While not contemning clarity (which, heaven knows, we all need more of), it tolerates a certain imprecision and irregularity in its ruminations about the moral dimensions of modern medicine. This tolerance does not arise from any perverse love of obfuscation, nor, I hope, from any neglect of sound logic. It comes, rather, from welcoming into the discussion of the moral dimensions of medicine the often obscure traditions of medicine's historical and mythic past. I happen to believe that ethical understanding comes as much from appreciation of tradition and history as from clarity of concept and rigor of logic. I feel it is important to strive for precision in discussions of ethics, but that striving should not be so strained as to eliminate the "variety and irregularity" of personal experiences, historical traditions, and cultural formulations. My friends, Tom L. Beauchamp and James F. Childress, have written a fine book, *Principles of Biomedical Ethics* (New York: Oxford University Press, 1989). They open with the comment, "We do not ignore the history of moral reflection in health care; indeed, we assume its relevance. But we emphasize the development of a theory and a set of principles for the treatment of problems that even the most elevated and ancient forms of medical ethics are ill equipped to handle" (p. 3). This book dwells on the "history of moral reflection in health care," in the conviction that its "elevated and ancient forms" may handle certain problems with a wisdom that theory and principle occasionally miss.

So this book attempts to accommodate the hard edges to the blurred outline. It watches the shaping of ethical questions through the long tradition of medicine in Western culture, a tradition that blends myth and history, science and philosophy. It seeks in that tradition an understanding of why we ask certain ethical questions of the new medicine. This is not a book of historical scholarship; it alludes to history. It is not a philosophical treatise; it refers to philosophical concepts. It is a personal reflection reaching for an insight into the encounter between the ethical tradition of Western medicine and the technological health care of today's world. This sort of rumination should not dull the sharp edges of medicine's technical skills, but only demonstrate that those skills can be most properly used when the "variety and irregularity" of the human condition in which they are employed is fully appreciated. To quote Aristotle again: "In medicine, it is easy to know what honey, wine and hellibore, cautery and surgery are, but to know how and to whom and when to apply them: that is truly to be a physician!" (V.9.1137a). Knowing how, to whom, and when—or, in Aristotle's other words, "what is appropriate to specific circumstances"—calls for a sensitive appreciation of the softer, less clear, often uncertain features of the human condition.

This book had its origins in an invitation from Harvard Medical School to deliver the George Washington Gay Lectures for 1988. Dr. Gay, a member of the Harvard medical faculty, founded the lectures in 1922, with the goal of promoting the education of medical students in "medical ethics and business." His linkage of two subjects today often considered antithetical is curious, but I am pleased at the thought that Dr. Gay must have been successful enough in his business to endow a lectureship that has lasted almost seventy years. Among the notable individuals in the fields of medicine and health care who have received the customary "modest honorarium" was Francis Weld Peabody, whose famous essay "The Care of the Patient" was the Gay Lecture for 1927. I am honored to be one of his successors. Dr. Daniel Federman, Associate Dean for Students and Alumni at Harvard Medical School, urged me to expand the Gay Lectures for publication. I am grateful to him for that suggestion and to Drs. Leon Eisenberg and Lynn Petersen, who were my gracious hosts during those pleasant fall days in Boston and Cambridge.

Contents

The New Medicine
and the Old Ethics

Introduction

Watching the Doctor

In some cultures, it is said, villagers cluster around a healer and a patient, eagerly listening to their conversation and observing their actions. In our culture, with its intensely private ways, we are deprived of this spectator sport. Very few are allowed to observe the intimacies of the "doctor-patient relationship." So in recent years certain persons—usually academic people, sociologists, anthropologists, economists, even philosophers—have arranged to watch from afar. They do not have a license to look and listen. Their justification is a discipline of some sort that claims that its methods and insights will somehow improve the relationship. So they watch from a distance (or sometimes only watch in their mind's eye) and write articles and books that describe, criticize, count, clarify, and occasionally complain. Our culture has transformed the fascinating pastime of doctor-watching into a science. We have elevated the gaping crowd into a bevy of professors and graduate students. We have orchestrated the ooh's and ah's into a critical literature.

I can hardly complain about all this, for I am one of those doctor-watchers. Decorated only with degrees in philosophy and in religious studies, I migrated into medical education, where I have been professing medical ethics for two decades. I follow the little party of doctors, nurses, and medical students to the bedside of very sick people. I read patients' charts, talk about patients' ills, participate in discussions about patients' fates. Although I eschew the pretensions of white coat and beeper, I admit to some gratification at being "inside." More than that, I believe that I have some right to be there and that my being there does some good to doctors and patients alike. I believe this because of the work I do.

My work is medical ethics. My professional title authorizes me to teach "ethics in medicine." I read and write about ethics. I have studied ethics, both as moral philosophy and as moral theology—two respectable academic disciplines that many people have never heard of. A while back, I was called to the chairmanship of a Department of Biomedical History, which on my arrival changed its name to Medical History and Ethics. I have always been interested in the history of medicine, and the privilege of associating with professional historians has enticed me further into that field. I cannot claim anything more than amateur status, but my attitude toward my own discipline has been colored by my dealings with historians. I find that I am now watching doctors with a bigger telescope: I see contemporary physicians as the latest workers in a long tradition. I see current ethical problems as new formulations of old problems. This book issues from reflections about the new medicine—the most up-to-date technologies and the most futuristic science—as it works within the old ethics, sensing ideals and constraints that perplex it and thrust it into ambiguities and paradoxes for which it is ill prepared.

As an ethicist, I am professionally concerned with ethical problems and the issues of the moral life. These can be found wherever human beings are found. (A competent article in a professional journal even explored the question of whether Robinson Crusoe had moral duties.) In medical care such topics abound: life-support systems, abortion, artificial hearts, genetic engineering, neonatal intensive care, research with human subjects, euthanasia. And these are only a partial index of the moral problems in medicine. In my daily activities I deal, in theory and practice, with these issues. But there is something else, something much more fundamental and interesting, that draws me to the ethics of medicine and to doctor-watching.

Having written these chapters, I was at a loss to know how to locate them in a recognizable literary genre. History they are not, although they relate some bits and pieces of the history of medicine and of the Western world. Philosophers would not recognize them as respectable philosophical discourse, although Aristotle and Jeremy Bentham and Alasdair MacIntyre show up from time to time. *Time* magazine and the *New York Times* serve up fragments of current events; the *New England Journal of Medicine* brings us up to date with medical science and health policy. Asklepios, a figure of myth and poetry, Jesus, a figure from revelation, and Sir William Osler, standing firmly in the annals of modern medicine, appear with equal billing. All of this is stirred together: what is the proper name for the potpourri?

While reflecting on this, I read a review of a new translation of the Talmud. The reviewer noted that most of the Talmud consists, not of *halakha*, or law, but of *aggadah*, "a magical rabbinic mode of thought in which myth, theology, poetry and superstition robustly mingle."[1] I had found my literary genre.

These chapters are secular aggadah. They move without embarrassment among myth, history, science, and philosophy, picking ideas and events that please. The excursion is not pointless, however; the ideas that are selected are bundled together in the hope that they will generate insight about the contemporary world in which physicians and patients meet each other. This world consists of more than encounters of actual people, of more than events statisticians can count, sociologists describe, and economists "cost out." It is really a world in which a very long history flows into current personal attitudes and institutional arrangements, in which the ideas and beliefs formed by myth and tradition are as powerful as the data of science and the provisions of policy. The moral life of that world cannot be delineated in clear, bright lines. It is rather a chiaroscuro in which shadowy figures from history, myth, and tradition are often more powerfully present than the pallid propositions of philosophical ethics. This is the world of medicine that I have been watching. My secular aggadah tries to describe its light and shadow, its foreground, background, and future.

Like the great panoramic portraits of the Flemish Renaissance, the figures and movements group around a central axis. In medicine's moral history and present, that axis forms at the point where altruism and self-interest meet. At that intersection a profound moral paradox pervades medicine. Certainly, every human being from time to time feels the tug of these conflicting motives, whether in personal life or in occupation. But it is my belief that the opposition is built into the very structure of medical care and woven into the very fabric of physicians' lives. The particular moral problems encountered in medicine are symptoms of this paradox. Many of the psychological troubles of physicians (and their families) are fomented by their inability to manage the pressures it generates. To be sure, I cannot support these assertions with solid epidemiologic studies or statistically impressive empirical research. I merely propose them as the reflections of a sympathetic and experienced doctor-watcher.

There can be no question that self-interest and altruism are elements in all moral life. They may even be seen as basic principles of the moral life. Some philosophers propose them as the only principles; others stress one principle at the expense of the other. Still others argue that one is a principle and the other an impulse that the principle must oppose. Regardless of how they are interpreted and combined, it is difficult to think about human morality without both traits. Self-interest is the principle that one should act so as to promote for oneself the values of preservation, growth, and happiness; even good done for others must redound to one's own good. Altruism is the principle that one should act so as to promote the preservation, growth, and happiness of other persons even to the detriment of one's own interests.

Philosophers would say, of course, that these definitions are overly simple. They are. Any perceptive person would see that they contain ambiguous terms. They do. And everyone can recognize that in daily life these principles are not mutually exclusive. Self-interest may rule most of our decisions and actions, but occasional generosity prompts true self-sacrifice. Some persons care deeply for others at great cost to themselves, but even they have moments of self-interest. Great moral lives are created out of the artistic harmony of both principles. We sometimes wonder whether even remarkable altruism is really only masked self-interest; we may, on the other hand, wonder whether self-interest has anything moral about it at all.

There is an impressive literature devoted to these fascinating and troubling issues. It is my thesis that medicine—as an institution, as a practice, as a profession—is dominated by the paradox in its starkest terms. There are historical, sociological, and psychological reasons for this. In this book I trace some of these reasons, using medical history and myth as well as moral philosophy to locate the new medicine in the old ethic, and to reveal the wisdom and the weakness of the old ethic in the face of the new medicine. I use history as a rank amateur, asking it to proffer exemplars of ideas rather than to interpret events. I unapologetically mix myth with history to convey the overarching, powerful, yet vague and somewhat mystical nature of tradition in medicine. I use moral philosophy lightly, asking it to be a source for reflection about crucial ideas rather than a tool for precise dissection of logic and concepts. From time to time, my text may turn a bit whimsical; for, as even the solemn rabbis of old knew, the most serious discussion can be advanced by an occasional smile.

This, then, is my secular aggadah. With it I hope to capture its own survival. The university must seriously respect the pursuit of truth; it is forbidden to censor, but it may rightfully expel barbarians who use "truth" as a weapon of destruction. The law feels the powerful strain of preserving the common good and at the same time ensuring justice to the individual. But its practitioners profess an ethic in the service of their clients, dominated by their communal self-interest. The American Bar Association affirms a rule of confidentiality that cloaks even ongoing crime. By a remote utilitarian calculus, this rule may possibly serve the common good, but it most assuredly serves the communal self-interest of lawyer and client. Remember, in submitting these reflections I am not accusing, condemning, or censuring; I am merely suggesting the way in which the weight and stress of moral principles are felt in institutions and by the moral persons who work within them.

Modern medicine inherits a long tradition in Western culture. Even today, when younger members of the profession know almost nothing of that history and when it seems fashionable to pretend that there was no history before antibiotics or before microbiology, the long tradition shapes medicine. There is a kind of moral archeology: digging beneath current moral beliefs, values, and practices, one discovers that these are built on ancient foundations not visible to the casual observer. The moral archeology of medicine exposes two traditions at the very deepest levels, one coming from ancient Greek medicine, the other from medieval Christian medicine. Scholarly studies of the Greek medical literature turn up precious little altruism in the ethics of the Hippocratic physician. Hippocratic medicine was a skill, its practitioners were craftsmen, and their objective was a good living. The etiquette that went by the name of ethics consisted of counsels of self-interest: "Act in this or that way with your patients if you want to build a reputation and a clientele." Even the beautiful phrase, "Where there is love of humanity, there is love of the art," which Sir William Osler extolled as the height of medical idealism, appears on close examination of text and context to be advice about good advertising. There was nothing unethical or immoral in all this; self-interest can be an adequate moral principle when safeguarded by the precept "At least do no harm." Not until the second century A.D., when Stoic and Christian ideals had a whisper of influence, did even a hint of altruism appear.

After some early distrust of medicine, the Christian church adopted care of the sick as a duty of charity. Sharing the Jewish theology of a God whose loving power heals through human instruments, the Christians added Jesus' parable of the Good Samaritan, who bound the wounds of a stranger beaten by thieves and had him cared for at his own expense. Monks and nuns became healers; the imperatives of self-sacrifice under which they lived were extended to their duties toward the sick and dying. They were admonished to remember the words of the Lord, "I was sick, and ye visited me . . . Inasmuch as ye have done it unto one of the least of these my brethren, ye have done it unto me" (Matt. 25:36, 40). Even in the ferocious Middle Ages, the Knights Hospitallers (or Knights of the Hospital), founded to care for those on pilgrimage and crusade, were commanded to treat the sick as "their lords." The Christian physician was obliged to remain in the plague-ridden city and to treat the poor without charge. There are parallel traditions in Jewish medicine. Medicine became Judeo-Christian, and altruism and medical care were bound in a moral covenant.

Both traditions still exist as the deep moral foundations of medicine. Medicine is a skill so rare that it can be sold at great price. Acquired with effort, it promises great rewards—not only of income but also of prestige, reputation, and gratitude. In this the modern physician inherits the Greek tradition. Nothing dishonest or shameful is involved, although, like any skill, it can be dishonestly and shamefully used. At the same time, medicine offers help desperately sought by persons often hard pressed to purchase it. They, and society, expect that the help will be forthcoming. Outrage greets stories of the uninsured injured who are turned away from emergency rooms; incredulity is the reaction when rationing of medical care is mentioned. Stories of the doctor whose golf game or cocktail party delays attendance at the patient's bed arouse anger. For the modern physician inherits the tradition of monastic medicine: he or she is servant to "our lords, the sick."

It is, I think, impossible for medicine to eradicate the traces of these ancient traditions. Even physicians who are indifferent to Hippocrates and have never heard of monastic medicine have these traditions stored deep in their consciousness. Society will not allow them to forget; society permits them to learn and use their skills in order to earn a living and, simultaneously, insists that those skills be used for the benefit of society. In order to safeguard this dual goal, Western society has invented the medical license—which, in the most peculiar way, reinforces the moral paradox of self-interest and altruism.

Licensure is, and has been since the late Middle Ages, a state's permission to practice medicine. For the last four centuries licensure has been surrounded by a philosophical and political conception, the doctrine of rights. The license confers a right to practice and creates a sphere of privacy and property over which the profession has close to exclusive rights. In most societies the organs of state have left to those skilled in medicine the right and duty to examine candidates and to supervise practitioners. Innumerable forms of this system have been developed, but in essence it has always come down to a social tolerance for a monopoly in return for a promise of social benefit in the form of competent and dedicated medical care. The monopoly exists because physicians set the standard of competence, educate the candidates, and examine their skills. Only those who meet the profession's criteria can reap the financial benefits of practice. On the other side, society demands that when medical skills are needed by its population, physicians must be prepared to provide them. Even when states do not guarantee medical care, they censure physicians who refuse to serve. In the United States legal reproofs are rare, confined almost entirely to situations in which abandonment can be demonstrated, but in other countries the responsibilities of physicians to render needed service are more stringently defined and enforced. Whenever concern over the inadequacy of medical care rises to the level of public debate, the underlying claim on physicians' skills also surfaces. Suggestions emerge about doctor drafts, mandatory practice in underserved areas, and national health services. Whatever the arrangements between society and the practitioners of medicine, the paradox of self-interest and altruism is reinforced.

This becomes apparent when the organized medical profession fears that its concerns are threatened. Its inevitable response is that the configuration favored by the profession is truly in the public interest. In the 1960s the American Medical Association opposed any form of national health insurance with slogans suggesting that government plans would destroy the incalculable social and personal benefits that patients experience when they pay for their own care. We now hear, from various professional groups, refutations of other proposed innovations: advertising will lure patients to quacks rather than to competent physicians; permitting patients to see their own medical records will frighten them; requiring informed consent will encourage them to reject appropriate procedures. Needless to say, arguments framed in this fashion may have some merit. But they need to be debated on their own grounds. My point here is that the self-interest of a licensed monopoly and the social promise of altruism live together in the profession's life. It is too easy to invoke one in order to dissemble about the other.

The paradox gets into the consciousness of physicians in another, more personal way. Insidiously and overtly, medical education encourages it. Young people enter medicine with a diversity of motives. At least as many come with strong altruistic ideals as come with hopes of earning a secure and lucrative living. Most, I am sure, come with mixed motives. In the intense competition for admission, in the incessant demand for performance in the laboratory, lecture hall, and ward, and in the renewed competition for desirable residencies, fellowships, or faculty advancement, all the intensity of self-interest is stimulated. At the same time, the altruistic ideals of the profession are proclaimed on every ceremonial occasion. Much more dramatically, the absolute asceticism of the residency recreates, for the young physician, the sacrificial ethic of monastic medicine. That ethic is severe: immediate response to the needs of the patient, to the calls of the emergency room, to the demands for reports; unmitigated responsibility for correct decisions made promptly and communicated clearly; the flagellating denial of sleep, self-indulgence, and frivolity, even to the point of depression and deterioration of personal life, friendship, and love. This practice, which is intense in the year of internship, must instill into many medical minds the monastic principle of altruism. Guilt is likely always to be felt in the future when a call is to be answered, a patient seen, or a consultation completed. The physician's conscience ever after will cry out when self-interest intrudes on patient care. At least, this seems to be the hidden rationale.

We hear reports of the high incidence of suicide, substance abuse, and marital failure among physicians. The harmful effects of stress, even if they do not break out in fulminant disorders, sap energy and enthusiasm. We all know personal stories of remarkable success in practice and disastrous failure in personal life. Despite psychiatric and social explanations of these phenomena, the answer may lie in the moral realm. Every physician in our culture must face the paradox of self-interest and altruism. No physician is permitted to be merely a profiteering tradesman; few bind themselves by vow to self-sacrifice. All physicians must live between these principles in institutions that enshrine both. The tension is incessant. Some escape by maintaining a charade of altruism; they become the covert medical businessmen. Very few physicians submerge all self-interest in unremitting service. Most attempt to maintain a precarious balance.

Along the fringes of the moral paradox appear those particular problems that we have come to call the ethical problems of medicine. These are of many sorts. Some are trivial but revealing, such as an exchange of letters in an influential medical journal about patients calling doctors by their first names. "Am I, who have worked so hard and learned so much, not deserving of respectful title?" says self-interest. "Do I not bestow my skill and learning with the loving generosity of a father to a child?" says altruism. Contrast this rather puerile case (which can, nonetheless, arouse indignation on both sides) with the much more serious debate that appeared in the pages of the same journal several years previously. Does the self-interest of physicians who have a financial stake in treatment centers impel them to provide medical services that are inappropriate for their patients and inefficient for society? "No," say the accused, "our services are measured to the real needs of our patients and provide important benefits to society." The ethical problems associated with the use of human subjects in research also bear the marks of the paradox: does the research procedure benefit the patient or promote the researcher's interests? A BBC documentary on medical research was titled, "Are You Doing This for Me, Doctor, or Am I Doing It for You?" Again, does the agonizing reluctance to discontinue life-support systems arise from a desire to give vitality to the patient or from the physician's fear of failure? All these problems have features of their own and must be analyzed and resolved on their own terms. Still, I suspect that the great structural paradox of medical morality runs deep within them all.

Let us suppose that my thesis about the paradox is true and that my description of its effects is accurate. Why should I be interested? I might have a speculative curiosity about the nature and consequences of an enigmatic morality; or I might have a morbid curiosity about the struggles of those caught in the paradox. I believe I do not have either, but rather have a practical curiosity. Is it possible to reveal to those who choose to live with the paradox its nature and consequences and to help them as they do battle with it? Can medical education be made more sensitive to the way in which it aggravates the paradox and more effective in preparing students to appreciate and tolerate it? Can institutional arrangements be revealed as products of the paradox, and can creative ways be found to ameliorate its crude and negative features? Can it be made clear to the profession and to the public that an honest acknowledgment of the tension could benefit all—that the tension itself need not be destructive but can strengthen personal life and community between physicians and patients? Can the conscience of the physician be instructed in the many specific ways the paradox will manifest itself in the course of practice and life?

These are the concerns that have motivated my teaching over the past twenty years and that motivate the presentation of this book. I believe that these issues can be illuminated, and their burden made more tolerable, by grounding them in the traditions of Western medicine. Let us, therefore, set off on a voyage through the history and myths of that tradition, a voyage that leads to today's scientific and technological medicine and pushes on into the future.

Chapter 1

Asklepios as Intensivist

In Seattle on March 9, 1960, Dr. Belding Scribner started to dialyze patient Clyde Shields. Dialysis is a medical technique whereby blood is passed out of the body, through a filtering machine, and back into the body. The external machine serves as a substitute for kidneys that are too damaged to perform their function of filtering impurities from the blood. For some patients, damage to the kidneys is temporary, resulting from trauma or poisoning. For others, damage is permanent and irreversible. Dr. Willem Kolff invented the dialysis technique in the 1940s, but it could be applied only for temporary relief of critical kidney failure; patients with irreversible and complete kidney failure inevitably died. Scribner hoped to keep Clyde Shields alive for a long time, because Shields could be dialyzed repeatedly through the new "Scribner Shunt" implanted in his forearm. After a previous patient, Neil Ward, had died because his successful dialysis could not be repeated, Scribner had awakened in the middle of the night with the idea of a permanent arteriovenous access—a tube that could be fixed into a vein and an artery, so that the patient could be hooked to and taken off the machine as often as necessary. Within a few weeks he and his colleagues had fabricated such a device from Teflon tubing. The shunt worked and Shields lived, with dialysis twice a week, for another twelve years.[1]

This event marks a suitable inauguration of the era of bioethics. We know full well that single events do not a historical movement make: the storming of the Bastille did not start the French Revolution any more than the "shot heard round the world" at Concord Bridge opened the American Revolution. Those dramatic incidents leap out of the long, slow accumulation of ideas, emotions, and activities that build into an identifiable "movement." The dialysis of Clyde Shields, or Belding Scribner's sudden inspiration to try a Teflon arteriovenous shunt for continuous dialysis, is for two reasons an appropriate moment to signal the start of bioethics.

The first reason is that the dialysis program to which that invention led quickly caught media attention. Within two years the Seattle Artificial Kidney Center had many more patients than it could treat. A method for selection of patients had to be devised. A committee of laypersons was asked to choose, from the many medically qualified patients, the few who would receive life-saving treatment. Shana Alexander told the dramatic story of the "life or death committee" in *Life* magazine.[2] The public attention stimulated scholarly reflection on the problem of "allocation of scarce medical resources," and the field of bioethics was born.

A second reason to choose a date in the history of chronic hemodialysis as the beginning of bioethics is that the problem of allocation of resources, while not the only problem of bioethics, is the paradigm for the most radical question that has faced medicine during its long history in Western culture. Bioethics has come into being, as a public interest and as a professional discipline, because medicine and health care face an issue that the traditional ethics of medicine had not previously faced and for which it had no ready response. The chapters of this book explore that new issue. We shall see the old ethics of medicine struggle with the new science of medicine; in that struggle the weakness as well as the wisdom of the old will be revealed. The task of bioethics is, in my view, to preserve the wisdom and to remedy the weakness, in the hope of formulating a new ethics to guide the new medicine.

It is common to trace the old ethics to Hippocrates, the Greek physician of the fifth century B.C. He and his disciples left a large scientific literature and a small collection of moral maxims. The former is now forgotten, although it dominated Western medicine for eighteen centuries; the latter remain in the collective memory of medicine. Hippocrates himself is a shadowy figure. Despite the fact that Aristotle called him "the Great Hippocrates," we know little about his actual life. But the origin of the old ethics can go behind the shadowy physician of history to a mysterious figure of myth.

Long before Hippocrates was born, stories were told about a demigod who was the patron of human healers: Asklepios, whose name appears in the oldest version of the Hippocratic oath: "I swear by Apollo, by Asklepios, by Hygeia, Panacea, and all the gods and goddesses . . ." He was, we are told in Greek mythology, the son of the god Apollo by the human woman Koronis. Indeed, the god extracted the infant Asklepios from his dying mother's womb, so that the procedure we now call cesarean delivery deserves the even more honorific title "Apollonian delivery." The god then entrusted the child to the centaur Chiron to be taught the art of medicine. The poet Pindar writes:

> He raised Asklepios, the gentle hero,
> craftsman in remedies for the limbs of men
> tormented by disease.
> Those who came to him with flesh-devouring sores,
> with limbs gored by sharp bronze
> or crushed beneath flung stones,
> all those with bodies broken,
> sun-struck or frost-bitten,
> he freed of their misery, some by the lull of soft spells,
> some by potions, others with bandages
> steeped in medication, and some he set right
> through surgery.

Asklepios was, in a sense, the first "intensivist," a forerunner of those modern physicians who respond to critical injury and insult with intensive, life-saving therapy. These are the physicians who preside over the intensive-care units. While modern intensivists have renounced the use of soft spells, they "set right" the badly damaged organs and limbs of those in danger of death. Asklepios' brilliant medical career came to a tragic end, however. Again Pindar tells the tale:

> Even wisdom feels the lure of gain—
> gold glittered in his hand,
> and he was hired to retrieve from death
> a man whose life was already forfeit to the gods.
> Zeus hurled flashing thunderbolts
> and drove the breath from both their chests,
> savior and saved alike.[3]

The fate of Asklepios did not mar his reputation. The guild of Greek physicians bore the name "Asklepiadae" and their places of healing, "Asklepieona." The dramatic ruins of several of these ancient clinics can be seen on the island of Cos (Hippocrates' home), at Epidauros, Athens, and elsewhere in modern Greece.

I have noted the resemblance between the work of Asklepios and the work of modern intensive and critical-care medicine. Obviously the resemblance is remote. Even more remote is the original moral of the story. Asklepios was struck down because he transgressed a divine decree; Zeus, jealous of his prerogative, took swift revenge. It mattered little that the ancient intensivist was bribed to his efforts; he worked to save a life already condemned by the gods. This is clearly a story of the very old medicine and the very old ethics.

But myth bears within its archaic forms perennial truths: there may be buried here a moral about the new medicine, which some ethical archeology can unearth. Certainly, Asklepios was described and remembered as a competent physician. He was the son of Apollo Physician and a student of the ingenious healer Chiron. He had all the skills needed for his medical and surgical work, and his success brought patients from all Greece. His competence, we can assume, would have saved the life of his condemned patient, otherwise Zeus would not have been so vengeful. So Asklepios was extending his competence into a forbidden field—life-saving service to one whose life was forfeit to the gods. Might we imagine that here the old story has a message for modern medicine, that perhaps there are fields forbidden to its competence? Ought medicine do everything it is competent to do? Strip away the divine prohibition and the tale speaks as much to the medical scientists, practitioners, and educators of the final decade of the twentieth century as it did to those who listened to Pindar's ode at Siracusa in 488 B.C.

The problem, then, is this: is there an ethical limit to competence? In one sense, ethics has always been about whether we ought to do what we can do. But for modern medicine it takes on a new meaning, because in this century competence itself has become the moral meaning of medicine. And at this point in the century the moral crisis of medicine concerns the limits to be imposed on competence.

Competence, in the sense of a disciplined understanding of the science and skilled manipulation of the art, has long been a medical virtue. If anything deserves the title "Hippocratic ethic," it is the imperative of competent practice of the art. Hippocratic writings do not use the word "competence" or any similar Greek words. Nonetheless, the essence of Hippocratic medicine was the insistence that "all disease has a nature and arises from a natural cause, and is capable of cure."[4] The Hippocratic physician was urged to "acquire true knowledge of medicine before traveling to various places and acquiring the reputation of being a physician in deed as well as in word . . . There are two things: science and opinion. The first begets knowledge and the second ignorance."[5] Hippocrates' *Precepts* makes the most definitive statement about competence in the context of condemnation of medical quackery:

> Conclusions that are merely words cannot bear fruit, but only those based on demonstrated fact . . . One must hold fast to

generalizable fact and occupy oneself with facts persistently, if one is to acquire that ready and sure habit we call the art of medicine . . . for to do so will bestow great benefit upon the sick.[6]

Thus, when the Hippocratic maxim is uttered, "Be of benefit and do no harm," and the phrase of the Hippocratic oath (probably not composed by Hippocrates) is sworn, "I will act for the benefit of my patient according to my ability and judgment," the imperative of medical competence is implied.[7] The physician is to know by evidence and logic the conditions that lead to disease and the remedies that can loosen its grip. The immoral physician is the one who exploits the patient's ignorance and vulnerability by the fiction of knowledge and skill.

When medicine was adopted as a university subject and a guild activity in the Middle Ages, competence became a notable and explicit virtue. In those settings the external elements of competence, namely subject matter on which to examine and peers to do the examining, became common. Competence consisted in mastery of the knowledge of those theories and observations enshrined in the thousands of pages of Galen, Avicenna, and other classical authors. The Royal College of Physicians of London examined this mastery by giving a candidate for licensure three random passages from Galen, shutting him in a room with an unindexed set of that author's works, and requiring him to find and comment on the passages! Another oral examination tested the candidate's knowledge of the "use and practice" of medicine. He was expected to know the conditions for purging and bleeding, the application of drugs, and the use and measuring of clysters.[8] The writings of the sixteenth and seventeenth centuries on the duties of physicians repeat as the first imperative, "Let the physician be competent." Roderigo a Castro's influential *Medicus Politicus* (1614) defines "physician" as *vir bonus medicinae peritus* (a good man expert in medicine), which is, ironically, a twist on Cicero's definition of a legal orator or lawyer. He then explains at length that one becomes *peritus* (expert or competent) by "sparing no labor to learn the truth about disease and healing."[9] A book by Ahasverius Fritsch, intriguingly entitled *The Sinning Doctor,* proclaims that the first mortal sin of physicians is "practicing medicine without being throughly competent in the art."[10] We may only hope, for their patients' sake, that their competence as healers extended beyond book learning!

In modern medicine, competence has become more than the first virtue; it is the essential, the comprehensive virtue. The etymology of the word, from the Latin *competere* (to seek or strive), suggests a drive, an impetus: the competent professional is not merely one who minimally qualifies, but one who seeks an ever more perfect understanding and performance of his or her work. Competence is a habit and, as philosophical psychologists from the time of Aristotle have noted, habits are performed with pleasure. Thus, the competent internist enjoys the intellectual act of differential diagnosis and selection of appropriate therapy; the competent surgeon enjoys the decisions and manipulations of resection and reconstruction—as surgeon-author Richard Selzer somewhere called it, "the handsomeness of the art." Further, competence creates a camaraderie of respect and appreciation among those who share the mastery of an art. Still further, competence inspires those who share it to expand it, for at the edge of every competency lies a challenge to enlarge its scope. Thus, competence in medicine implies the inspiration of the practitioner, the unity of the profession, and the impetus of the science.

Competence needs something objective to hold to and be measured by. Modern medicine has provided that handle and that measure by evolving in this century into a discipline dominated by objective data. Medicine is the physiology and pathophysiology, the immunology and microbiology, the genetics and neuroscience, that deliver a factlike, quantifiable picture of order and disorder within the body. Correspondingly, competence consists in the comprehension of these data as they are appropriate to a specialty, and their application to particular instances. Competence shows itself in measurable ways: its methods and achievements are open to objective evaluation in ways that have never before been possible in medicine.

This is now so much the case that the nonobjectifiable features of medical practice are pushed to the periphery. The so-called humanistic virtues are treated as ancillary to the central core of competence, which lies in mastery of data and method. Alternative theories that attempt to expand the vision of the physician, such as the "biopsychosocial" approach, linger on the outskirts of "serious" medicine. Lacking strong objective warrants (the so-called hard data), these theories fail to flourish in the modern climate. There is an old canard that always brings smiles and nods: "I'd rather have a competent bastard do my surgery than a bumbling humanist."

The centrality of competence to the ethics of medicine was first emphasized at the beginning of the twentieth century by a distinguished member of the Harvard Medical School faculty, Dr. Richard Cabot (1868–1939). The medical historian Chester Burns has written of Cabot as follows:

> By the fourth decade of the 20th century, the American medical conscience had been reshaped . . . The all-purpose general practitioner of the 19th century—a Christian gentleman of intrinsic goodness, law abiding and loyal to the codified rules of one professional society—had been replaced by a new group of specialist practitioners . . . rooted in experimental science and elaborate methods of clinical evaluation and patterns of clinical care . . . As much as any other physician of his day, Richard Cabot demonstrated the validity of the new bases for professional goodness . . . Whether or not the practitioner went to church on Sunday, knew the "Star Spangled Banner," swore the Hippocratic Oath, or adhered to precepts about consultation in the AMA code of ethics were not the important criteria for judging professional propriety. What counted [for Cabot] was whether a practitioner understood specific diseases, their causes, signs, symptoms, courses, prognoses, treatments—and whether each practitioner applied this understanding in the assessment and management of each individual patient.[11]

Cabot, who concluded a distinguished career as professor of medicine by holding a Harvard chair in social ethics, had caught the spirit of turn-of-the-century medicine. It was a medicine excited by the explosions of knowledge in pathology, pathophysiology, and bacteriology and progressing rapidly toward more factual nosology and diagnostics. These scientific advances informed a new ethic of competence. It was the primary duty of the physician to know and use this information in the care of his patient.

Clinical competence, Cabot felt unequivocally, must include not only mastery of science but appreciation of the personal and social needs of the patient. Like his younger colleague Francis Peabody, Cabot understood and taught that the "care of the patient is in caring for the patient."[12] He recognized what we now call the humanistic qualities of the physician not as mere decorations on clinical competence, but as intrinsic to it. The fact that we are still worried about the absence of humanistic qualities and still trying to discover methods of educating students in them reflects their recalcitrance to objectification, not their essential function in competent clinical practice.

The ethics of competence, fully understood as mastery of the science and skills of diagnosis, therapy, and prevention of disease, together with an appreciation of the personal and social aspects of the patient's health and disease, are the glory of modern medicine. They are the standard to which all physicians must be held—the goal of medical education and the expectation of the public. These ethics of competence might well be given the eponym "Cabotean ethics," since Dr. Cabot did so much to articulate them. They can stand as the modern extension of Hippocratic ethics into the age of scientific medicine.

Cabot's modernized ethics of competence may look like the

new ethics for the new medicine. And, indeed they were, for fifty or sixty years after Cabot formulated them. They are, however, starting to look as antique as the therapeutics Cabot knew as a clinician. Appropriate for the scientific medicine that emerged in the second half of the nineteenth century, they are challenged today by a new science and by new social problems. Sad to say, the Cabotean-Hippocratic ethics of competence are the "old ethics" of the title of this book. As they face the new medicine at the end of this century and the beginning of the next, they are ethics in crisis.

The ethics of competence not only imposed the imperative to understand thoroughly and use correctly the science and art of medicine, they also required an appreciation of the limits of competence. Competence is, without doubt, a virtue; yet, as Aristotle pointed out so long ago, by defining virtue as a mean between extremes, competence can fail by lack or by excess. The lack of competence in physicians was the most prominent problem of nineteenth-century American medicine: Cabot and others were dedicated to the eradication of *incompetence*. Yet competence can be excessive: skills can be overused, or used in the wrong place and time for the wrong purpose. Thus, as Cabot and his colleagues inculcated competence, they also had to discover the limits of competence.

Again, we should not be surprised. Morality often poses barriers to competent action. Police who can competently extract confessions are morally forbidden to do so. Soldiers who certainly can competently kill civilians are morally restricted from so doing. We might call this the Patton or MacArthur problem: these were two very competent generals whose competent military judgment suggested that they press on to Moscow or Beijing, but whose competent judgment was overruled by extrinsic political considerations, decisions made by persons whom the generals considered incompetent. Our question, then, is, What should be the limit, or limits, of competent medical action?

Earlier, I noted the remote similarity between the activities of Asklepios and modern intensive-care medicine. That rather lighthearted comparison can be translated into a serious statement of my case. Intensive-care medicine is a remarkable development of the past thirty years. The concentration of technology to manage acute cardiac, respiratory, and renal failure and to counteract the lethal effects of multisystem organ failure requires significant science, skill, and precise, rapid organization of information and response. Intensive care is undoubtedly a paragon of competence in care of the patient.

It is also an arena for ethical problems. Most of the familiar cases of modern medical ethics—Quinlan, Fox, Dinnerstein, Brophy, Herbert, and the series of Baby Does—were played out in intensive-care units before they went to the courtroom. In these cases the problem was not incompetence; the skills of diagnosis and treatment were unquestioned. The wife of a patient whose irreversibly unconscious life was being sustained against her wishes complained, "It's not that he's being poorly treated—he's being *too well treated.*" In each instance the question was, Is this competence rightly used or are there limits to competent medicine? A vast literature of legal and ethical commentary has explored this question and, to some extent, reasonable answers and acceptable policies have emerged.[13]

Broadly speaking, the intrinsic moral limits of medical competence have been recognized: the patient's refusal of further assistance, either entirely or in some particular respect, and the physician's recognition that further assistance will be ineffectual in improving the patient's condition. The undesirability and the futility of further medical attention, combined in various ways, underlie the ethics of withdrawing or withholding competent care. These are ethics that fit the fashion in which medicine has developed over the last century. They set moral restraints on the excesses of the virtue of Cabotean competence.

Yet Cabotean ethics are themselves becoming old, for we are on the edge of a new medicine that will challenge their assumptions in peculiar ways. The new medicine just coming into being differs from current medicine in that its science is population based rather than patient based. The Cabotean ethics of competence focused on the correct use of diagnosis and therapy for the presenting patient. This will, of course, continue, since the object of medical attention will remain the care and cure of a presenting patient. But in the emerging medicine the presenting patient, more than ever before, will be a representative of a class, and the science that makes possible the care of the patient will refer prominently to the population from which that patient comes.

From the time of its nineteenth-century beginnings, modern medicine indisputably has been a population-based science: diagnostics and therapeutics have grown out of studies anchored in statistics. But those populations have been the background of an intensely patient-oriented medicine. The emerging medicine draws those populations into the fore-ground. In specialty after specialty the genetic bases of disease are being revealed. One day, as I was composing this chapter, the front page of my *New York Times* headlined, "50% of Colo-Rectal Cancers Tied to Genetic Predispositions."[14] Several weeks before, a short article had reported the claim that the genetic basis for schizophrenia had been identified. We now have the capability of ascertaining the onset of Huntington's disease before its dread symptoms have shown themselves. The mapping of the human genome will track more and more clinical entities to specific sites on the human chromosomes, which means planting these diseases in the prolific garden of the human population. We have long known, for example, that diabetes was an inheritable condition; we now know that a gene on chromosome 6 accounts for 50 percent of genetic susceptibility to insulin-dependent diabetes. We had not clearly known that rheumatoid arthritis was a genetic condi-tion; we are now aware that a collagen gene on chromosome 6 may effect connective-tissue disorders. Can prenatal or pre-symptomatic interventions for diabetes, arthritis, and a host of other conditions be far behind?

The potential for genetics and molecular biology to reveal the populations apt to be affected by disease is obvious. In another field of the emerging medicine, transplantation, the patient is also surrounded by others—those who are likely donors of organs and tissues (relatives, accident victims, or aborted fetuses). A young mother recently underwent the haz-ardous donation of a lobe of her liver so that it could be implanted in her two-year-old who was dying of biliary atresia. As in the growing list of genetically based diseases, where the potential victims are the population at large, so in transplantation the potential saviors are the population at large. In yet another area of the emerging medicine, disease prevention, populations move to the foreground; for the key to prevention of cardiovascular disease, certain cancers, substance abuse, and so forth, is behavior change at the level of populations.

To be sure, medicine has always faced the problem of disease in populations. Containment of epidemic disease and prevention by immunization belong to the old medicine. But the new epidemic of AIDS has recalled with horrifying vividness the links between individual illness and the health and disease, behavior, knowledge, and values of populations. The discomfort we feel over the conflict between protecting the uninfected and respecting the rights of the infected is a manifestation of our strong commitment to a patient-centered ethic of competence as it faces our looming awareness of a population of infected persons dwelling in a population of infectible persons. In this vision, the patient-centered ethic is threatened.

Even in intensive-care medicine, there is interest in delineating the characteristics of patients so as to determine which patients are statistically more likely to benefit from intensive care. A growing number of studies attempt to specify the probabilities that a certain medical intervention will yield a certain outcome and, conversely, reveal the conditions under which the probabilities for success are low. One of those systems bears the evocative name APACHE (Acute Physiology and Chronic Health Evaluation)—intensive-care units are known for their "aggressive care," just as Geronimo was known for his "aggressive" defense of Amerindian lands. Should the perception that a given patient, with an APACHE score of 30, has a less than 10 percent chance of survival justify the decision not to admit that patient to the intensive-care unit? In other words, should a statistical expression of probability serve as an intrinsic limit of competent medical action? This patient is viewed as representative of a population. Should his or her physician relinquish the absolute dedication to this patient—who is, after all, a statistic of one?

And so it goes. The science of medicine, in one area after another, reveals more clearly than ever before that *this* patient, with *these* signs and symptoms, represents a population. Medicine is learning to intervene in various populations, by testing, by warning, by behavior change, by transplantation, by genetic diagnosis and therapy. One might play on words by saying that medicine is moving, in its knowledge base and in its practice, from intensive to extensive, from an intensive concentration on the presenting patient to an extensive awareness of the population behind the presenting patient. The competent cardiologist of today who has mastered, for example, the equations relative to myocardial oxygen consumption will be replaced in a decade by the cardiologist who knows in addition, with equal precision, the ratios of HDL to LDL that will, in the words of Cecil's *Textbook of Medicine,* "clearly identify those in the population who are at especially high risk of cardiovascular disease." [15] The competent oncologist of today has mastered the complexity of combination chemotherapy regimens; his successor will profit from the fact that, in the words of Nobelist Michael Bishop, "the long imagined cancer genes have been brought to view . . . and we have laid hold of cancer with a grip that should eventually extract its deadly secrets" [16]—secrets written in the human genome, with the possibilities of diagnosis and prevention at the genetic level.

Thus, in one after another of the conventional specialties and their sciences, the patient will be drawn into a population, seen as heir to or progenitor of disease, or as participant in a pool of risk. It may be that now, 150 years after the German pathologist Rudolf Virchow's prediction, medicine is about to become a "social science," not merely because its activities take place within the limits and potentials of society, but because its very base in biochemical knowledge testifies to its social dimensions. [17]

The drift of medicine from a patient base to a population base poses a major challenge to the ethics of medicine, ethics that have grown up around the imperative of competence in patient care. The intrinsic ethical limits to competence, based on undesirability of care from the patient's viewpoint or futility of care from the physician's, are no longer sufficient. Even if a particular patient should judge medical attention to be undesirable, we know that others in the relevant population may be affected by that refusal or need information or therapy that depends on the patient's decision. Some of those others may not be identifiable or even currently extant: the fetus of a pregnant woman who rejects the abortion option despite an inheritable disorder, or the son of a man with Huntington's disease who declines testing and goes on to procreate. Even if a particular intervention may be futile in assisting one specific patient, it may be of benefit to some other—as in the case of the brain-dead mother perfused for two months to bring her fetus to viability, or the anencephalic perfused until his heart and liver can be transplanted into another baby. Competence now extends beyond the care of the presenting patient. Should the ethics of competence require medical attention to individuals other than the patient?

The new medicine begins to present, in scattered fashion, problems that the old ethics Hippocratic and Cabotean, find puzzling. The dilemma comes not from their being new problems, but from their being without roots in previous ethics of competence. Almost all the ethical problems faced by the old ethic could be resolved within the framework of a relationship between the professional and the patient; the ethical problems posed by the new medicine reflect the omnipresence of the population that stands behind that relationship. This is not to say that those problems are insoluble, but only that their resolution calls for a perspective unfamiliar to Hippocratic and Cabotean medicine.

It is now possible to see why Belding Scribner and Clyde Shields, on that March day in 1960, opened a new era for the ethics of medicine. Shields was a chronologically first patient; he was symbolically the precursor of a population of patients. In the case of dialysis, that population was the class of patients with end-stage renal disease that soon appeared on the doorstep of the Seattle Artificial Kidney Center and within a few years were lobbyists in the antechambers of congressional hearing rooms. The plea of that population was to "provide us with financial support so that we may benefit from the treatment that your scientific competence has made possible." As a result of congressional action in 1972, amendments to the Social Security Act provided financial support for renal dialysis and transplantation (our American form of organ-by-organ national health insurance). But another ethical problem arose thereby: the problem of the limits of competence. Now that we can provide dialysis to all patients in medical need of it, should we? Are there patients who, because of age or other medical problems, should not be treated? The best endocrinology and nephrology does not have an answer to that question. It belongs to bioethics.

Remember the fate of Asklepios. He transgressed a limit set not by his competence, but by Olympian ordinance. Aristotle, who was the son of an Asklepian physician, must have known Pindar's tale of Asklepios' tragic end. In a paragraph of his *Nicomachean Ethics*, Aristotle almost seems to recall the demigod's story:

> To know how actions must be performed and distributions made in order to be just is a harder task than to know what makes men healthy. It is rather like medicine, where it is easy to know what drugs, cautery and surgery are but to know how to administer them, to whom and when, in order to make the patient healthy, is the truly difficult task of being a physician.[18]

Poor Asklepios did not know "to whom and when" his competence should be applied. Although the physician with Cabotean competence may sometimes be uncertain how and when medical skills should be applied, he is quite sure to whom—namely, the presenting patient. The physician of the new medicine will not even be sure of that.

"To know how actions must be performed and distributions made in order to be just," says Aristotle. Let us consider whether the new element in the ethics of competence must be justice, a virtue that has never been prominent in medicine.

Chapter 2

The Good Samaritan as Gatekeeper

Some years ago two leaders of American medicine, Walsh McDermott and David Rogers, published an article in which they made a plea for "samaritanism" in modern medical care. By this term they meant the "human support function . . . that eases the acceptance of technology and allows it to be applied . . . to temper the harshness of illness." [1] McDermott and Rogers refer to the parable told by Jesus and recorded in the Gospel according to Luke (10:29–37, King James version):

> But he, willing to justify himself, said unto Jesus, And who is my neighbor? And Jesus answering said, A certain man went down from Jerusalem to Jericho, and fell among thieves, which stripped him of his raiment, and wounded him, and departed, leaving him half dead. And by chance there came down a certain priest that way: and when he saw him, he passed by on the other side. And likewise a Levite, when he was at the place, came and looked on him and passed by on the other side. But a certain Samaritan, as he journeyed, came where he was: and when he saw him, he had compassion on him, and went to him, and bound up his wounds, pouring in oil and wine, and set him on his own beast, and brought him to an inn, and took care of him. And on the morrow when he

departed, he took out two pence, and gave them to the host, and said unto him, Take care of him; and whatsoever thou spendest more, when I come again, I will repay thee. Which now of these three, thinkest thou, was neighbor unto him that fell among the thieves? And he said, He that shewed mercy on him. Then said Jesus unto him, Go, and do thou likewise.

The parable of the Good Samaritan was used in the first centuries of the Christian era and throughout the Middle Ages to exemplify the duties of the Christian physician. In particular, the tale reinforced the duty to care for the needy sick, whether friend or enemy, even at cost to oneself. The early Christian writer Saint John Chrysostom, recalling the parable, commented, "It matters not whether the sick one is Christian, Jew or Gentile, it is his need that calls out to you."[2] Even though this lesson was originally preached when monks and nuns provided much of the care for the sick, it has persisted into our secular era as a principle of medical ethics. Modern physicians are most certainly not copies of Mother Teresa, but they are, in moral tradition, her spiritual relatives. We recall the principle, even if not the parable, when we discuss the responsibility of physicians toward the indigent and toward persons with HIV infection. This "Samaritanian principle" deserves to stand beside the "Hippocratic principle" of competence in its importance for medicine in our culture. The medical historian Henry Sigerist wrote that from the time Christianity spread and became the religion of Western society, "the duty of society to care for the poor and the sick was never disputed, even when it was not fulfilled."[3] Thus, two broad ethical traditions flow through Western medicine: competence and compassion. The ideal physician has always been seen as the bearer of both virtues, and departures from either have been deplored.

But more can be drawn from the parable than the picture of the compassionate physician and the principle of service to those in need. A parable, like a myth, stimulates our imagination to see in ancient words a modern problem. For us that problem is summarized in the title of this chapter. The gatekeeper designation encompasses one aspect of what philosophers call the problem of justice in the allocation of scarce health-care resources.

Let us return to the parable and do some imaginative exegesis. Saint Luke is reputed to have been a physician, and there is the slightest suggestion in the text that the Samaritan was a healer or physician: technically correct words from the vocabulary of ancient medicine are used for "bandaging the wounds," and infundation of oil and wine was a standard therapy for open wounds, mentioned in the Hippocratic literature and elsewhere.[4]

Assume, then, that the Good Samaritan was a Samaritan physician committed to the principle that the needy sick should be cared for regardless of economic status, racial identity, or political affiliation. Encountering a person in serious need of medical service, this physician readily responds. Suppose, however, that as he transports the comatose patient to the nearest hostelry, he encounters another victim of the bandits. His little donkey can carry only one burden. The second victim is seriously wounded, not half dead, and perhaps more likely to survive than the first. The Good Samaritan is faced with a problem of triage.

Deciding on a first-come, first-served rule, he leaves the second victim and continues on to the hostelry. He stabilizes the patient and turns him over to the innkeeper for nursing and rehabilitation. He pays the charges himself and, recognizing that this patient may be what our current Medicare payment system describes as an "outlier" (a patient whose care will cost more than the set reimbursement), says he will reimburse any additional cost. The Good Samaritan, at this point, is very much like the primary-care physician in a contemporary "managed-care system." He is referring the patient to another "provider," and the cost of the additional services may be charged to the referring physician's allocation of funds and the income of the health-maintenance organization of which he is a member.

The Samaritan physician continues his journey, heading to visit some regular, paying patients in nearby villages. As he travels, he finds even more victims of the brigands and discovers that even his regular patients have been impoverished by their pillaging. Now he realizes that he will not be able to recoup from his paying patients the costs he might have incurred by taking responsibility for the wounded traveler. Indeed, few of his patients can any longer pay for his services. Yet all are in need of medical attention and he is committed to the principle of service to the sick.

Throughout these events the priest and the Levite who had "passed by on the other side" are still standing back. They had ignored the wounded man, contrary to the injunctions of the Jewish law, which imposes a duty to help the sick based on the words of the Book of Deuteronomy, "and thou shalt restore it to him"—a phrase originally pertaining to the return of lost animals and later applied by rabbis to the task of restoring health.[5] The two religious functionaries had avoided the wounded traveler, even though he was "their brother"—one of their own faith—possibly because they feared he might die during their ministrations to him and thereby pollute them by contact with a corpse, strictly forbidden to the priestly caste. Thus, contrary to the teachings of most rabbis, they put their ritual purity before their duties of charity. Two of the many paintings of the scene, one by Jacopo Bassano and the other by Vincent van Gogh, show the clerics walking away with their nose in a book, perhaps seeking a legalistic justification for their blatant neglect of the duty to help. They watch the Samaritan doctor struggle with the disaster. Less concerned about their ritual purity than about the solvency of the temple's treasury, they are willing to dispense a few shekels here and there, for decency's sake, but hardly enough to meet the need. As to the innkeeper whose inn is converted into a hospital, he is a generous fellow, but after all he has a business to run.

Perhaps this fantasy overplays the parable, but we can extract from it a moral that fits our present-day problem. This Good Samaritan represents the good physician of today. He has the essential virtues: the Hippocratic-Cabotean ethics, which prohibit exploitation of patients and demand competence, and the Samaritanian ethics, which enjoin compassion and non-discriminatory service to those in need. His quandary, with more sick persons than he and his friend the innkeeper can care for, is how to distribute his resources of time, energy, and money among all who can benefit from his attention, now and in the future. He wonders how he can be not only a competent but a just physician, giving to each his or her due.

Justice in health care is the leading topic of medical ethics today and is being considered by many fine scholars. Yet, these elaborate philosophical discussions, important though they are for a general comprehension of the problem of allocation of resources, may fail to address the dismay of the 1990 Good Samaritan. How, he may ask, can I be a *just* physician or, more seriously, is it even possible to be a just physician in an unjust system? Can there be a just health care in the United States?

Some years ago, the dean of the Harvard School of Public Health, Howard Hiatt, wrote an important essay, "Protecting the Medical Commons." [7] That article was among the first to declare that rationing of health care was inevitable. Dr. Hiatt proposed, however, that any rationing be done not by practitioners, whose first allegiance must be their patients, but by policy makers, who were removed from direct responsibility for individual patients. In the fifteen years since Hiatt wrote that essay, his appreciation of the moral responsibility of the physician has been challenged by major changes in the policy, financing, and institutional arrangements of health care. Hardly a physician today is immune from the demand to ration, whether that demand comes in the mild form of cost-effective ordering or in the extreme form of explicit restrictions on availability of services or referral. Indeed, the decisions of the physician dealing with the patient are the primary rationing device.

In recent years the word "gatekeeper" has designated the role of the primary-care physician who is charged with directing patients through the system of specialty referrals in the most cost-effective manner. Lately that metaphorical term, with its Dantean implications, has been replaced by the more anti-septic "case manager"; but the earlier metaphor is a more striking expression of the ethical problem. Many forms of gatekeeping have been devised, particularly in so-called man-aged-care systems. Almost everyone, proponents and oppo-nents, recognizes the potential for conflict between patient advocacy and institutional cost control, a conflict that can result in the twin evils of underutilization and overutilization, the first to the disadvantage of the patient and the second to the detriment of the plan's pocketbook.[8]

Scarcely a physician today has failed to experience some conflict between the principle of service to the sick and the solvency or profitability of the institution or practice in which he or she works. Allocation of resources is not only a philo-sophical problem of justice, not only a political problem of health policy; it is—or should be—a problem of conscience for the practitioner. To what degree can the old ethics meet the new medicine to resolve that problem?

The Hippocratic, Cabotean, and Samaritanian principles do not quite reach the issue of justice. They have not considered the question of who among all potential patients has the right to the services of physicians. The old ethics spoke to physicians about their actual patients. Justice in health care has no actual patients: it seeks a principle of distribution that will, in antici-pation of actual need, count some persons as worthy of atten-tion and count others out. From this viewpoint the line at the clinic extends infinitely. Each patient whose name is called is immediately replaced by another. Should a principle of distribution be found, it would allow the intake nurse to drop certain designated persons out of the line or to pull certain designated persons from the back to the front. To anyone who complained, she could cite the principle of distribution: "Sorry, but it is fair and just."

It is common to say that we must employ the principle of triage to select patients for scarce resources. But triage, taken from its context, is an empty principle. The French word means picking and choosing. French railroad workers know that the term *voie de triage* means a siding and *gare de triage* means a marshaling yard. Anyone who has spent a Saturday night in the emergency department of a city hospital will appreciate those expressions. But the question remains, What determines the picking and choosing? Originally the principle was clear. Baron Dominique Jean Larrey, surgeon general of Napoleon's armies, is credited with using the term to designate the practice of battlefield medicine. As a continuous stream of wounded are carried toward the surgeons' tent, they are laid out in order of arrival. A surgeon walks among them and picks out those who can be most quickly treated and restored to the line. Speedy restoration of fighting function is the objective. The more difficult cases wait, regardless of the seriousness of their need.[9]

Theologian Paul Ramsey pointed out some years ago that the principle of military or disaster triage has a clear objective: to save the most salvageable so that they can contribute to the common good—which, in the battle, is victory; in earthquake or fire, is public safety. The common good provides the criterion for selection.[10] When triage is taken out of that clear context, it becomes little more than using French to say, "We've got to make a tough choice." It offers no guidance in how to do so. Indeed, in Saturday night emergency department triage, General Larrey's principle is reversed: the most seriously wounded are rushed in and the merely mutilated must wait.

Our story of Dr. Scribner and his patient, Clyde Shields, illustrated the problem that brought bioethics into being: Who shall be saved when all cannot be saved? Within two years of Shields's dialysis, the pressure of the multitude of patients with end-stage renal disease (estimated—indeed, underestimated—at that time to be sixty thousand to eighty thousand in the United States) forced the Seattle Kidney Center to answer that question in a practical way. A committee of laypersons was formed and asked to choose from the many medically suited candidates those few who would receive dialysis. Their triage needed a new principle: there was no battle to be won, no devastated city to be evacuated.

No amount of reading in the codes of ethics, no deep reflection on the Hippocratic, Samaritanian, and Cabotean ethics, could turn up a suitable principle of triage. The Seattle Committee, unfairly nicknamed the God Committee, did its best without formal principles. It utilized some commonsense maxims: younger rather than older patients, those with dependents rather than those without, the emotionally mature and stable, those with a record of public service, and so on. Before the committee went out of existence, rendered unnecessary by congressional enactment of legislation that provided federal funding for patients with end-stage renal disease, all of these maxims had been subjected to severe criticism. Philosophers, theologians, and lawyers, who did not themselves have to make the selections, came up with "better" approaches. The earliest books and articles on bioethics were filled with studies on the ethical and legal problems of selection of patients.[11] Then, for a few years in the mid-1970s, the newborn bioethics neglected (except as academic exercise) the problem that had given it birth. Selection for hemodialysis had been ended by government largesse, and the philosophers seemed satisfied that their analyses had demonstrated that random selection by lottery was ethically superior to the crude and discriminatory "social worth" criteria that appeared to govern the Seattle Committee's painful deliberations.

Still, the problem of allocation of resources did not disappear. In the early 1980s it returned with a vengeance. Americans realized that medical care was costing a great deal and that many people could not afford it. We discovered, much to our surprise, that Medicare and Medicaid had large gaps and that 35 million Americans (that was the generally accepted figure in 1980; it has grown since then) had no health insurance or had inadequate and sporadic coverage. The problem of allocation could not be resolved by lotteries: some form of rationing seemed imperative. The Good Samaritan was perplexed, not by how to select patients for a single new intervention, but how to get care for all who needed care. A bigger and better triage principle was needed to supplement the Hippocratic, Cabotean, and Samaritanian ethics. Today's Good Samaritan can call on the bioethicists for help. For their part, the bioethicists are busy studying what has now become a full-blown problem of distributive justice.

Despite the hard thinking of the bioethical scholars, I doubt that any satisfying principle of triage or rationing will be devised. My skepticism arises not because I am impressed by philosopher Alasdair MacIntyre's thesis that no "neutral, impersonal, tradition-independent standards of justice" are rationally viable.[12] My skepticism about a principle of distribution in health care rests on more narrow grounds. I wonder whether the work of medicine is in fact compatible with *any* strong theory of justice. I am inclined to agree with the late Paul Ramsey, who wrote that the "larger questions of ordering our medical and social priorities are almost, if not altogether, incorrigible to moral reasoning."[13] Can the institution of health care be equitable in its essential features of access and quality? Can the compassionate Samaritan be a just Samaritan?

The first issue, usually designated that of "macroallocation," is concerned with the fair distribution of burdens and benefits throughout the health-care system. It worries about whether the elderly or the young deserve greater access, whether primary care or major rescue interventions, such as organ transplantation, deserve priority. It faces the pleas for support of different sectors of society: education over health, defense over education, and so forth. The macroallocation problem is a philosophical one, but it is also a problem of health policy and politics. It is, for better or worse, in the hands of the modern successors to the theocratic priests and Levites of the parable, and they are rarely inclined to listen to Samaritans or philosophers.

The second issue, often called "microallocation," deals with choices among patients with particular afflictions or particular characteristics under conditions of scarcity. It is a problem of philosophy and a problem of medical practice. Microallocation challenges practitioners in the daily work of deciding how to allocate their energies to patients and in the task of determining how the institutions in which they practice will distribute available services. The problem of microallocation in the office, in the clinic, and in the hospital creates another radical challenge to the old ethics of competence, analogous to the one we saw in the first chapter. There I suggested that the new medicine, being built on an emerging scientific base of molecular biology and genetics, presents a new problem to the old ethics of competence—namely, how to think about obligations to one's patient in relation to the populations that are beginning to appear behind the presenting patient. We can see the intense concentration on the presenting patient expanding into an extensive awareness of the others who are directly implicated in the patient's disease and treatment. This poses a significant and troubling question for the ethics of competence: Who is the patient?

The Samaritan, too, committed to the ethics of compassionate response to need, looks up from a single needy patient to a population of potential patients, an infinite line at the door of the clinic. The Samaritan is aware that time, attention, and money devoted to the patient now in his arms may mean that the next victim of the brigands will have to lie unattended. His essential ethical problem is not whether to serve his own interests rather than those of the patient (he has already settled that by prior dedication to samaritanism), but whether to serve this patient so completely that future patients may be excluded from attention. The Good Samaritan as gatekeeper must be sure that the gate is never permanently locked, but is opened and closed to admit all the needy in a timely and orderly fashion.

In terms of clinical decision making, this sort of gate-keeping must have its rules. The old ethics offer some advice. Cabotean ethics of competence have important implications for reasonable rationing. They rule out the gross moral abuse of omitting clearly indicated tests, procedures, and referrals in favor of the physician's or the institution's profit. Thus, the ethics of competence do provide a primitive rationing principle: each patient who comes into care must be treated in accordance with the standards of competence. The practice, the plan, the hospital, the system should accept only those patients who can be properly treated—and no more.

Even the Good Samaritan found that his charity had its ethical limits: the strength of his donkey, the availability of bandages, and the supply of oil and wine in his flasks. He would have acted inappropriately had he taken on more wounded than he could properly care for. His first patients would have suffered because he could not attend to them; his new patients would have received inadequate care. All the patients would have been harmed. The Samaritanian principle cannot be fulfilled by violating the Hippocratic rule to do no harm or by skimping on Cabotean competence.

We see that Cabotean ethics exclude undertreatment and forbid inadequate treatment. They also have a stronger imperative: do not overtreat. Overtreatment is as much a mark of incompetence as undertreatment. In the distant past unethical surgeons were accused of surreptitiously keeping wounds festering so that the patient would continue coming for care; unethical physicians falsely used their principal diagnostic technique, inspection of urine, to find disease that was not there. These practices were designed to prolong patient dependence unnecessarily. Today overtreatment is more elaborate and less obvious. Among its forms might be included persistence in attempting and continuing interventions that have very low probabilities of benefiting the patient. Under the guise of "doing everything possible," procedures of decreasing probability are dramatically and desperately applied. The reasonable judgment of futility is erased by therapeutic enthusiasm. The distinguished Harvard surgeon Francis D. Moore commented on certain dramatic organ transplantations:

> We often read in the medical literature that some patient was so desperately ill that almost anything was welcomed by the patient, the family and the physicians. This sort of hyperbolic "desperate remedies" pressure on physicians and patients should be looked on with skepticism. There must be some likelihood of success before the desperate remedy becomes more than a desperate search for an opportunity to try a new procedure awaiting trial.[14]

So even within the Cabotean ethics of competence, despite their lack of a rule for choice of patients, there is an implication for rationing of care: the absolute exclusion of useless interventions and the prudent use of those with little likelihood of benefit. Within these constraints it is ethically praiseworthy to acknowledge futility, improbability, and unlikelihood.

Futility and improbability are ambiguous words. They refer directly to the statistical chance of attaining a result and indirectly to the quality of the result itself. Given the power of technology, effects are produced with some regularity, but the effects are often dubious benefits. The premature infant is pulled through the crisis of respiratory distress syndrome and left with a terribly damaged brain. The victim of myocardial infarction is resuscitated but left in a persistent vegetative state. The implanted artificial heart "works" for two months, providing a life of unremitting crisis, distress, and dementia.

Here Hippocratic ethics make a contribution to the modern problem. They allow for consideration of the quality of even probable successes. Hippocrates is said to have belonged to the sect of Asklepiadae priest-physicians. In his *Republic* Plato wrote a miniature treatise on medical ethics in which he relates that the Asklepiadae repudiated any form of treatment that did nothing but "pamper disease." Asklepios, he says, "exhibited the power of his art only to persons who, being generally of healthy constitutions and habits of life, had a definite ailment; these he cured by purges and operations and bade them live as usual . . . But bodies which disease had penetrated through and through he would not attempt to cure . . . The art of medicine was not intended for their good." [15]

We are rightly wary of allowing "quality of life" judgments to determine who should be treated medically and who should be cared for in other ways. Yet the obligation to use medical skills, in the Hippocratic tradition, arises from the benefits the patient will experience as a result. "I will act for the benefit of my patient according to my ability and judgment and do no harm or injustice," states the oath. Even more pointedly, the Hippocratic essay entitled "The Art" says that the work of medicine is to "lessen the violence of disease, relieve pain and avoid attempts to cure those whom disease has overcome." [16] The injunction to bring benefit requires a serious evaluation of the quality of health and life restored; the injunction to avoid harm and injustice requires that we reflect whether some forms of continued life constitute an injustice, an unfairness to the one who must live that life. Many medical interventions succeed in giving burdens to the patient without compensating benefits. The President's Commission for the Study of Ethical Problems in Medicine heard the distant echo of that tradition when it proposed that only "proportionate" treatment is obligatory: treatment that promises more benefit than burden to the patient. [17] These are perilous and difficult considerations, prone to distortion by prejudice and ignorance, yet modern medicine must face them. When prudently employed, they become a principle of rationing within the Hippocratic tradition.

Cabotean ethics of competence can reduce expenditure of effort on the futile and improbable. Hippocratic ethics of avoidance of harm bid us refrain from medical successes that are nothing but burdens to the patient. Neither instructs on how to think about the line of persons waiting outside the clinic door, the infinite file of individuals who will become patients in the future. Physicians traditionally have employed a kind of rough moral rule of thumb, accepting patients first come, first served; patients who fit their specialty; in emergencies, patients in serious, immediate need; and in times of disaster, patients according to the rules of triage. The Samaritian virtue of compassion dictates some such approach, inasmuch as it is unable to tolerate the obscene spectacle of the sick and wounded lying untended. It goes further, seeking out the sick lying deserted by the roadside and bringing them into care. It dictates that one work harder, stretch one's efforts to accommodate more needy, and even accept financial loss if necessary. In the past, when simpler modes of financing prevailed, medicine maintained the Samaritanian principle of care for the poor by shifting costs between paying and nonpaying patients. As the medieval surgeon Henri de Mondeville wrote, "Treat the poor for the love of God, but make the rich pay dearly." [18] Modern methods of paying for medical care by third-party payers render this form of "occult compensation" obsolete. Still, the impulse of Samaritanian ethics pushes the good physician beyond the realm of practice into the world of policy. A bold approach to the authorities is required, to the priests and Levites in a theocracy, to the legislators, administrators and regulators in a democracy, asking them, Is this a society we can be proud of? a society in which the sick and the wounded lie unattended? Can you not find the shekels to insure all, or at least those who cannot pay? In modern terms, this means that physicians have a moral obligation to promote those forms of health service and health insurance that will encompass the largest number of persons. These ethics reprehend the self-interest that prompts professions to protect those institutions and arrangements that profit themselves.

The old ethics, then, do not lack sage advice about the new problems raised by gatekeeping. They advise: Do not admit a patient who cannot be given competent care; never omit a clearly necessary procedure for an admitted patient; do not employ technologies of unproven efficacy; stretch your capabilities as far as possible without compromising competent care. Behind these rules, a deeper problem lies. It is hinted at by the use of words such as "clearly necessary" and "unproven efficacy." The clinician's judgments are always in the realm of probability; they are calculations of prudence, not of mathematical science. Hardly any procedure is known to be absolutely necessary or unnecessary; hardly any technology is proven to be absolutely efficacious or inefficacious.

Thus, the essential moral problem of gatekeeping concerns the degree of certitude required to judge a procedure necessary or efficacious. This is not a new concern of medical ethics, generated by modern technology and statistics. Ethicists of the sixteenth and seventeenth centuries, called and unjustly maligned as casuists, expended much thought on the degree of probability or certitude required for responsible moral judgment. They did not, of course, mean probability in today's statistical sense, but instead the likelihood of performing a morally right action in a specific case. In situations of profound moral importance they frequently required what they called the *via tutior*, the more safe course. In applying this rule to practical cases, they insisted almost unanimously that when a physician was in doubt about the efficacy of a treatment he must choose the safer course; even a remote possibility that a treatment would save a life made that treatment mandatory. This rule of the casuists equals in stringency the rule of the rabbis commanding the preservation of life. [19]

The old moral rules of the casuists and the rabbis still echo in the subconscious or in the superego of the modern competent physician. They dictate "Treat rather than don't treat" and "Test rather than don't test." They are enunciated in the frequently stated but often statistically silly "3 percent or 5 percent chance of pulling through" that prefaces a decision to "go all out." They underlie the skepticism with which so many physicians view the methods of cost-benefit analysis, the invocation of quality of life related to clinical outcome, the suggestion that this or that intervention is of only "marginal" benefit.

I propose that the good Samaritan can be a just Samaritan only by adopting a less stringent rule of moral probability than those inherited from the casuists and the rabbis. While the old rules are good ones when one wounded person is under our care, and when one threatened life might be saved, they falter under the pressure of many threatened lives, of long lines of wounded and sick. The less stringent rule would require not taking the most safe way, but a probably safe course. Cabotean ethics require rigorous evaluation of therapies, a technique that modern medicine is only now learning to perform in theory and has far to go in applying to practice. Dr. Marcia Angell has suggested that more careful attention to evaluated efficacy is the rationing technique appropriate to the physician: it is in essence a combination of Hippocratic and Cabotean principles, avoiding harm by competent clinical judgment.[20] In contrast to rough guesses that went by the elegant name "prognosis" during most of medicine's history, physicians do have data that can inform their assessment of probabilities. The data are, admittedly, still crude and certainly incomplete, but the ability to classify disease patterns, to evaluate diagnostic and therapeutic interventions, and to identify outcomes in relation to interventions is immeasurably greater than in the past. Current studies provide useful information about the efficacy of certain critical procedures such as cardiopulmonary resuscitation, admission to intensive-care units or to burn units, and even about the utility of less critical procedures such as the probing, thumping, and listening done in routine physical examinations.

All such studies produce statistical data. Rarely can it be shown that a generally accepted intervention yields 0 percent benefit; more frequently, a small fraction of patients will benefit from an otherwise inefficacious procedure. For example, less than 5 percent of patients with an APACHE score of 30 can be expected to benefit from admission to an intensive-care unit; 3 percent of patients with metastatic disease survive cardiopulmonary resuscitation for at least twenty-four hours. The old *tutiorist* rule requires the physician to apply a procedure that offers any chance of saving life. A more relaxed rule would allow the selection of a level of probability or a reasonable chance. It would remove from the moral vocabulary of medicine the phrase "Do everything" and substitute "Do as much as is reasonable."

Naturally, the term "reasonable" evokes eyebrow raising and the inevitable cynicisms "Whose reasonableness?" and "What's reasonable?" Still, reasonableness has a reasonable reference, namely, the honorable traditions—Hippocratic, Samaritan, Cabotean. Taken together rather than singly, they point toward more comprehensive ethics that can accommodate both allegiance to one's patient and justice to all who will be patients. The three sets of principles that have made up the ethics of medicine converge toward the ethics of justice. The Samaritan recognizes persons in need. The Hippocratic enjoins only those treatments that are effective and beneficial. The Cabotean can make an informed decision about the nature and extent of that need and the means to remedy it. Together they point to the justification for a shift of moral probabilities from the absolute "Do everything possible for this patient" to the proportionate "Do everything reasonable for all patients."

This shift of moral probabilities is justified not by cost considerations as such or by any other social utility. It is justified as justice: not in the sense of some single principle of distribution, but in the sense of a moral disposition in the practitioner. This is Aristotelian justice, "a state of character which makes people disposed to do what is just, makes them act justly and wish for what is just."[21] This disposition inclines the competent practitioner to treat each patient with as full a range of resources as is compatible with the capability of other unknown and unseen patients to receive treatment when their time comes. It deprives no patient of genuinely needed care; but that need is now viewed not only as a pathophysiological state, but also in the light of the patient's quality of life and the burdens borne by those closest to the patient. It allows a broader probability for failure, not because this patient is worth less than any other, but because other patients are as worthy as this one. Finally, in an imperfect world where all resources, actions, and possibilities are bound by finitude, the just man must still, as Aristotle said, "wish for what is just."

This line of thought is fraught with hazards. It raises questions about the nature of clinical information and clinical judgment. It raises the threat of misuse of quality-of-life criteria and social utility. It challenges the primacy of patient autonomy and recalls the specter of physician paternalism. Even more, it imposes upon the practitioner of medicine and the philosopher of medicine the obligation to become much more definitive, in theory and practice, about the nature of medical need and medical intervention. It means that practitioner and philosopher must redefine, but not abandon, the traditional ethic of advocacy for the patient. That redefinition would lead to what might be called proportional advocacy, whereby every patient is not merely *this* presenting patient but *all* potential patients, and whereby the advocacy argues not for "everything possible" but for everything "probably beneficial." It is the task of the discipline of medical ethics, in the next phase of its work, to investigate and analyze these ideas, and the task of medicine to incorporate whichever of these ideas pass conceptual muster.

The good Samaritan can be a just Samaritan, giving to each his or her due, recognizing that behind each presenting patient awaits another patient in need of service. Even in a system of unjust distribution of resources, the practitioner can effect justice in small circles, as it were. A famous physician of the sixteenth century, Giovanni Codronchus, advised his colleagues, "If a physician has many virtues, yet lacks justice, all his other virtues, or most of them, will certainly fail him, for justice is the sum and source of all virtue." [22] He could not have been thinking about gatekeeping in a managed-care program, but modern gatekeepers or case managers would do well to

Chapter 3

The Nobility of Medicine

"Ethics" and "ethos" are twins in the family of words. Descended from the same Greek word meaning custom or habit, they are difficult to tell apart. Yet over time they have developed rather distinct connotations. "Ethics" designates the variety of rules, principles, and virtues that make up the moral life and, more particularly, names the philosophical study of the moral life. "Ethos" refers to the characteristic spirit and beliefs of a community or society, which may include, but is not limited to, its ethics. Ethics cannot be understood without ethos. All rules, principles, and virtues, while they may be stated in propositions and definitions, have a tone and color different in different communities. The principle of autonomy, to take an example popular in modern bioethics, may be given the same definition by American and by French moral philosophers, but the spirit and sense of autonomy will be quite different in Paris than in San Francisco.

An ethos is, in a sense, the climate in which ethics lives. Ethical rules and values take on a certain shading in light of the ethos. In recent years the ethics of medicine and of health care have been much discussed; the ethos of medicine and that of the medical profession have been less examined. Certain current ethical problems may be better understood if the ethos behind the ethics is made more explicit. I reflect in this chapter on an ethos that has had a powerful effect on medicine and on its practitioners—the ethos of nobility. As in previous chapters, historical persons and institutions will serve to make vivid the abstractness of the ethos. We begin with one of the true noblemen of modern medicine, Sir William Osler, founding faculty member of the Johns Hopkins Medical School and later Regius Professor of Medicine at Oxford.

On June 22, 1911, the Saturday morning mail brought to the Osler home in Oxford a confidential letter from 10 Downing Street, London. The missive bore the news that Dr. William Osler had been named baronet on the occasion of the coronation of King George V. Although Osler was unquestionably the most distinguished physician in English-speaking countries, the honor was a surprise to a man born in the genteel poverty of the Canadian countryside and comfortable with the vigorous democracy of Canada and the United States, where he had spent most of his career as a medical educator. Several days later Dr. Osler wrote to a friend, "They have put a baronetcy on me—much to the embarrassment of my democratic simplicity—but it does not seem to make any difference in my internal sensations." [1]

One month later Sir William spoke in Reading, a few miles from Oxford, at the unveiling of memorials to the first and last abbots of the great medieval monastery of that city—an uncharacteristic appearance for the Regius Professor of Medicine, but one to which he had been enticed by a physician whose hobby was the history of the abbey. In his address the new peer said: "You see here in stone symbolized the beginning and the end of a great epoch—of a vast movement to the strength of which our wonderful cathedrals and many other superb ruins bear enduring testimony. Marvellous, indeed, was the faith that found expression in such works! Small wonder that the thirteenth has been called the greatest of centuries." [2]

Sir William, in accepting the baronetcy despite his "democratic simplicity," stepped into a medieval tradition. He became a knight, a peer of the realm. He accepted a title and a few prerogatives (though only a few) that came to him from one of the most powerful social institutions of our culture, the knighted nobility, an institution that came into being throughout Europe as the Roman Empire fragmented into innumerable duchies and baronies and counties, served by men sworn to fealty to liege lords.

William Osler, physician, scholar, gentleman, by his sovereign's will became a knight. Certainly Sir William did not identify himself with the customs, ideals, and concepts of the vanished class. Indeed, by speaking of his democratic simplicity, he repudiated them. He graciously accepted the empty honor, long shorn of its political and military might. Despite his remark on the occasion of the Reading Abbey ceremony— he was quoting the title of a book by a friend, physician and historian James J. Walsh, *The Thirteenth, Greatest of Centuries* [3]—Osler probably had little esteem or love for that era, over which still hung the cloud of the Dark Ages. He called it, in a letter to Walsh, "a wretched, out-of-date community." [4] Sir William was, above all, a classicist of antiquity and the Renaissance. There is no evidence in his writings that he was particularly familiar with, or fond of, the Middle Ages.

In fact, we can imagine that he, like many of his contemporaries, found something rather extreme, rather grotesque, in the Gothic.

His entry into the titled nobility is more a symbol than a significant fact about Osler's life and thought. Sir William was a peer of medicine rather than a peer of the realm. He came to prominence as a physician in the last decades of the nineteenth century, a time when a number of medical men had achieved notice among their colleagues and before the public—a notice that paid homage to scientific learning and healing skills but, more than that, to the creation of a distinctive profession in the modern sense. Educated in universities, authors of scholarly volumes, influential in public affairs (particularly in the relatively recent public health reforms), founders and promoters of the relatively new public hospitals—these men formed a kind of nobility. They were, in skills and in science, persons of account. As Osler himself said, they made medicine "a profession of cultivated gentlemen." [5]

Many of these peers of medicine had been knighted: Sir Arthur Keith, Sir Thomas Lewis, Sir James Mackenzie, Sir Ronald Ross, Sir Thomas Allbutt—whom Osler's close friend, medical historian Charles Singer, called "the most learned physician of the last 100 years" [6]—and above all, the great Lord Lister, Baron of Lyme Regis. In democratic America, Osler had left behind an untitled peerage of equal prestige: William Stewart Halsted, Oliver Wendell Holmes, William and Charles Mayo, Walter Reed, William Henry Welch, and the young man who would become his biographer, Harvey Cushing. Sir William and his contemporaries brought to the medical profession a respect it had historically lacked. It still enjoys the trailing clouds of glory.

These peers of medicine also were nobles in their ethics toward their patients. While it is difficult to know with certainty, both because the record is not written and because the motives of men cannot be easily read, their lives and writing leave the impression that their ethics were "noblesse oblige." Although we use this phrase with disdain today, it has a noble history. It recalls the moral obligation placed on lords to protect their vassals, or on knights to protect the poor and the weak. Power, coming ultimately from God, was to be used for God's favored poor; fealty to a liege was reciprocated by the liege's duty to protect the vassal. These were ethics perhaps more honored in the breach, but they represented an ideal that created civilization out of chaos.

Noblesse oblige can designate a moral attitude or disposition that reflects, even at great distance, the knightly ethics. It describes the attitude of persons brought up in a definite tradition, enjoying privileges of social status, wealth, and education and endowed with a strong sense of their own worth and dignity. Essential to the tradition is the doctrine, religious or secular, that the privileges are not earned, but bestowed. They are given by divine grace or by good fortune of birth. Those who enjoy them must do so in gratitude, and gratitude is best expressed by doing good for less fortunate others.

Many of the renowned physicians of the late nineteenth and twentieth centuries seem to have ascribed, even unknowingly, to these ethics. The medical men of the eighteenth century were, by and large, a disreputable lot. Regular practitioners were poorly educated and often dishonest. Leaders of the profession, such as the Fellows of the Royal College of Physicians, were contentious and haughty. In the late decades of the eighteenth century, however, the status and education of doctors began to improve and the image of the gentleman-physician began to appear. The opening words of the paradigm book of medical ethics, penned by British physician Thomas Percival in 1803, bear witness in elegant language to the ethic of noblesse oblige:

> Physicians and surgeons should minister to the sick, reflecting that the ease, health and lives of those committed to their charge depend on their skills, attention and fidelity. They should study, in their deportment, so to unite tenderness with steadiness, and condescension with authority, as to inspire the minds of their patients with gratitude, respect and confidence.[7]

These words were incorporated into the Code of Ethics of the American Medical Association and stood unchanged from 1847 to 1912; their spirit lived long after that.

The writings and lectures of Sir William Osler do not discourse at length on the duty physicians owe their patients. His view was quite simple and straightforward. He once stated that, as part of his personal moral creed, "my second ideal has been to act the Golden Rule, as far as in me lay, toward my professional brethren and toward the patients committed to my care."[8] What we might call ethical problems are almost unseen in his voluminous writing. He does inveigh against ignorant doctors and polypharmacy, but there is nothing like, for example, the elaborate reflections on truth telling by his younger contemporary, Richard Cabot of Harvard, whom we have met before in these pages.[9]

Osler everywhere evinces an appreciation of the Hippocratic obligation "to be of benefit and do no harm." He was also committed to Cabotean ethics before Cabot stated it: a strong dedication to clinical competence based upon science. His whole career as practitioner, scientist, and educator bore witness to that commitment. As he once wrote, "To track to their sources the causes of disease, to correlate the vast stores of knowledge, that they may be quickly available for the prevention and cure of disease—these are our ambitions."[10] In addition to his commitment to scientific medicine, Osler's life and writings reflect an attitude of courtesy, respect, and kindness toward patients and colleagues. One has the impression of a dedication to the cure and comfort of the sick, even when it entailed, as it often did, a measure of personal risk. Sir William represents the ethos of medicine more than the ethics: one can sense in him an attitude and a dedication, even when there is little evidence demonstrating interest and knowledge of specific ethical issues.

Osler was a mirror for physicians of his day and of many decades thereafter. He himself, as he said of certain senior colleagues, "exemplified those graces of life and refinements of heart which make up character."[11] Physicians educated in the English-speaking countries during the first half of the twentieth century were conscious of their privilege: the profession had achieved social respectability and its education was vastly improved. Its practitioners had a sounder and sharper understanding of disease than their predecessors; they possessed some genuinely effective therapies. They could expect to earn a good living; at the same time, they were aware of their ethical duties toward their patients and of their philanthropic duties toward the sick poor. Unremunerated service in the public hospital and unpaid teaching in the medical school were mandatory.

The "old boys" of this era are still with us. Every medical society and medical school knows them. For the most part retired now, they are distinguished in mien, sober in dress, courteous, discreet, of curious intelligence, and—interestingly—either quite conservative or quite liberal in their political sympathies. They speak with gratitude of their teachers and with nostalgia of the simplicity and the rigors of their days in practice. They are men (almost always men) who, in Osler's words, "combine a stern sense of duty with the mental freshness of youth."[12] For the doctors of their generation, privileged in training and in respect, ethics are noblesse oblige.

The ethics of noblesse oblige, despite their somewhat antique formulation and dated sentiments, are unquestionably noble. They are rigorous in their demands and gracious in their effects. Those who lived by them did much that was beneficial. It is difficult for anyone to criticize them without seeming either cynical or so morally fastidious as to be foolish. Still, there is a flaw. It will not appear while the social conditions that bred the ethos remain stable. But when social conditions change markedly, the defect can be disturbing and perhaps even fatal. The flaw is the strong tendency of the nobility to defend itself and its privileges when under attack.

Even the most generous and benevolent noble can withdraw into the manor under the onslaught of the "ungrateful."

The nobility of Sir William and others of his ilk has a historical antecedent. It can be traced to an era in medicine's history when nobility and knighthood flourished more vigorously than in the England of Osler's baronetcy, a time when knights deliberately pledged themselves to be healers and servers of the sick and poor.

Sir William probably knew of the Knights Hospitallers of Saint John of Jerusalem—indeed, he may have been inducted as a member of their modern remnant, the English Priory, a largely honorary group that still maintains an Ophthalmological Hospital in Jerusalem and sponsors Saint John's Ambulance, an emergency transport service in England. In light of his general disinterest in the medieval era, however, he probably paid little attention to the history of that religious-military order and knew little of its practices.

Founded in Jerusalem at the end of the eleventh century, the original purpose of the Knights Hospitallers was to provide hostels for pilgrims to the Holy Land and to care for the sick among them. Its members were vowed religious, with obligations to celebrate the divine office in choir and to live in celibacy and poverty. Most were from noble families and were designated knights according to the practices of chivalry. They were trained to nurse the sick, and some of them were physicians. At Jerusalem, Acre, and other places on the route from Eastern Europe to Palestine, the order established institutions that were precursors of the modern hospital. The famous hôtels-dieu, more immediate predecessors of today's hospitals, were modeled on the Hospitals of the Knights of Saint John. [13]

Within a hundred years of its founding the order had assumed military duties as well, for it became obvious that the routes of pilgrimage needed to be protected against Muslim incursions. Many local Christian rulers deeded frontier castles to it and, despite its youth, the Hospital became a mighty military force, assuming political power in Cyprus, Rhodes, and Malta. Members of the order never abandoned their care of the sick, but this work of mercy became subordinate to the vast military and naval apparatus. The infirmaries are but a small section of the immense fortresses whose ruins still can be seen in the Near East. These religious knights, sworn to nurse the sick, became knights in fact as well as in title, and in the course of time the virtues of religion apparently were over-whelmed by the power and glory of military life.

Still, to the end of the reign of the Knights Hospitallers (which came at the fall of Malta to the Turks in the mid-sixteenth century), the brothers maintained their dedication to hospital work: it remained the soul of their community. Every brother at his induction recited the vow found in the earliest rule of the order:

> The brethren of the Hospital should serve our lords, the sick, with zeal and devotion, as if they were serfs to their Lords. (Rule of 1181)

Furthermore:

> How should our lords, the sick, be received and served? When the sick man shall come to the hospital, let him be received

thus: let the Holy Sacrament be given him and afterwards let him be carried to bed and served there as if he were a lord. (Rule of Blessed Raymond, c. 1150)

Centuries later the leaders of the Hospital continue to proclaim:

We make a promise which no other people make, promising to be the serf and slave of our lords, the sick. (Chapter of 1301)

The rule bears witness to this dedication in many ways: the sick were to be served their food before the brothers, were to eat off silver plates, were to be given white bread, were to have first call on bedding.

Our lords, the sick, shall each have their own sheets and coverlet, broad and long, as well as a gown and slippers to go to the latrine.

Our lords, the sick, who die in the hospital, if they have shirts and breeches, shall be buried in the same. (Chapter of 1301)

The revenues that supported the Hospitals were not to be diverted to other purposes. In 1296 the officers of the Hospitals complained that the Masters had been spending improperly the resources "that should have been spent for the benefit of our lords, the sick, to sustain them and the poor." [14]

Many of the brothers left the chapel and rode off to war, where they killed and maimed, as did all other knights. Some, like other churchmen corrupted by money and power, made a mockery of their vows of celibacy and poverty. Yet in those words, "our lords, the sick," they left medicine a precious heritage. They introduced, in antique language, the obligation to serve the sick regardless of risk or cost, a duty unknown to Hippocratic medicine.[15] They placed themselves at the command of those whom they treated; they subordinated, in principle, their ease and their convenience to the patients whom they received into the Great Hospitals at Jerusalem, Acre, Cyprus, and elsewhere. The parable of the Good Samaritan spoke to the Knights with great eloquence. They transformed the Gospel text "he had compassion on him" into a way of life. The wounded traveler became lord over the one who nursed him. To this the Knights vowed their lives.

It is important to realize the meaning, to a medieval man, of an oath "to be the serf and slave of our lords, the sick." The Knights of the Hospital, often born and bred of the nobility, well knew the social position of the serf. The serf simply had no rights and many onerous duties. Will Durant lists seventeen obligations of the serf to the lord, ranging from taxes in money to days of labor in corvée and even including the infamous *jus primae noctis,* in which the serf's right to sleep with his bride had to be redeemed by money. While in fact, as Durant says, the actual life of the serf may not have been as terrible as we imagine it, it was defined in terms of obligations and not at all in terms of rights.[16]

Thus, in a kind of pious irony, the Knights inverted the ethos of nobility. The noblesse oblige of chivalry, in which the knight and the noble had duties because they had received favor and grace from above, became the moral obligation of one bound to a master. Nobility consisted in the power to serve, not in the right to be served. This ethos was, of course, inspired by the Gospel in which they fervently believed; for

Jesus, Lord and Master, said to His disciples, "I am among you as one who serves" (Luke 22 : 27). Just as He chose to transform his divinity into the state of servant, they voluntarily transformed their knighthood into servitude. Thus their ethos was one of dedication to service. It lingered through the subsequent centuries. The first Code of Ethics of the American Medical Association (1847) opens with the words, "A physician should not only be ever ready to obey the calls of the sick, but his mind ought also to be imbued with the greatness of his mission and the responsibility he habitually incurs in its discharge." [17] That noble injunction was deleted in the 1912 revision of the code. Nonetheless, today, after the theological sources of this ethos have faded and its codified expression has been expunged, it remains a strong motivation for health professionals, many of whom have never heard of, or believed in, its theological origins.

The concept of nobility is so antiquated that it seems strange to recall it in the context of modern medicine. Is there any value in suggesting that modern medicine ask itself whether its practitioners are a peerage in the fashion of Sir William and his colleagues, or a nobility like the Knights of the Hospital? Is this a foolish proposal? Why should modern physicians think of themselves as a peerage or a nobility at all? Is not such a metaphor outmoded, even outrageous?

It should not be dismissed too quickly. First, the profession is still held in high honor, even though its prestige has slipped. Second, it is still a profession bound by an obligation to competence and to service—it alone among the professions still honors an oath. In these features it is somewhat like a nobility. But even more, it is held to act in concert as a barrier, a wall of protection, against the ravages of illness in individuals and in society. In this it acts as the medieval nobility, as protector of the realm and of the people. Osler recognized these duties, saying, "The physicians' challenge is the curing of disease, educating the people in the laws of health and preventing the spread of plagues and pestilence." [18]

Nevertheless, the flaw of the noble ethos may be affecting the ethos itself. We have seen that nobles, capable of generosity when in power, retreat into protective positions when under attack. They hold power and bend gratuitously to protect the poor. Yet having never relinquished power, they can readily become inaccessible by raising walls of stone, or of costs. In this is the modern lesson. The nobility of medicine has, in the last century, attained great power: the profession's monopoly has created great institutions and controls a vast economy. Its control lies not in the sword but in the prescription. But in recent years, that power is being eroded by the government, by insurance companies, by the courts, and by legislators.

In the next chapter we will hear a physician complain that medicine and physicians are "beleaguered," a word that means "camped around" or "under siege." It is an image that recalls the history of nobility, created to defend the realm, and of the Knights Hospitallers, building fortresses to protect their patients and pilgrims. Today, of course, the besiegers are not the Turks but government regulators, utilization reviewers, malpractice lawyers, third-party payers, and even patients. As a cover story in *Time* put it:

> The air of the operating room, where once the doctor was sovereign, is now so dense with the second guesses of insurers, regulators, lawyers, consultants and risk managers that the physician has little room to breathe, much less heal. Small wonder that the doctor-patient relationship, once something of a sacred covenant, has been infected by the climate in which it grows . . . Ambivalence and hostility divide doctors and patients. [19]

The "sovereign" doctors and the "sacred covenant" of this paragraph of mixed metaphors are remnants of the old nobility of medicine. As present-day medicine begins to feel embattled, will it fight, as the Knights of the Hospital did when the power of the Turks moved against their holdings? Will it turn, as did those same nobles, from protecting the poor to protecting itself and its status? Will the modern knights of the hospital rally to defend their powerful fortresses, as did the Knights of the Hospital at the siege of Malta? It is all too easy to defend power and prestige by claiming that they are needed so that the poor can continue to be served: if the fortress falls, the infirmary within it will close. The ethos of noblesse oblige falters when the power of the noble is attacked. It is a powerful ethos only when it adherents are safe. Even in its benign form, it is in essence an ethos capable of being dominated by self-interest.

The original dedication of the Knights of the Hospital to

"our lords, the sick" was quite different. It saw the relationship not as a spillover of power, a trickle-down ethic, a condescending compassion flowing from power, but as a comprehensive commitment of energy to those who have no energy. In this view, institutions are constructed to empower the powerless. Those who build and guard them must be dedicated to this goal and keep vigil over themselves lest they turn the institution to their own ends. They must be willing to make personal sacrifices so that the work of healing and helping can go on. They must be ready, when the institution is threatened, to rally around their sick charges rather than around their treasury.

The siege of modern medicine comes from another quarter, and it is more ominous than the guerrilla incursions by regulators, administrators, and litigants. It is the massing army of persons unable to afford medical care. In the United States health insurance has become the primary means of payment. Doctor and hospital bills are paid by insurance companies or by the forms of public insurance called Medicare and Medicaid. Yet in 1989, 37 million people, or nearly 18 percent of the population, have no medical insurance. Of these, 18 percent work full-time for employers who do not provide insurance benefits; 15 percent more work part-time. Less than 13 percent earn annual incomes under $10,000; the majority of the uninsured, almost 50 percent, make as much as $30,000. Some of these individuals get no health benefits from their workplace and are unable to afford private coverage. Others have health conditions that make them uninsurable.

Others, with assets that make them too "wealthy" for public assistance, are too poor to insure themselves; they receive no medical attention until crisis brings them into public hospitals. All these 37 million persons are outside the fortress of modern medicine.

The siege they mount is not a physical one: they are not pounding battering rams at the gates. They may not even be angry about their plight. Their siege is a moral one: they challenge the noble ethos more poignantly by their very presence than by violent attack. Noblesse oblige and dedicated service motivate the physician to care for those sick who ask for care. They even urge exceptional efforts to keep open the doors for those who seek care. But this noble ethos is baffled by the prospect of large populations that are, it seems, disenfranchised. They rarely have the means to approach for care and, when they do come, they are rebuffed by institutional barriers that are dropped only when ability to pay can be demonstrated.

In the past, the ethos of nobility dictated its own conditions for service. Today, those terms are set by external institutions. Treatment must be given in hospitals, drugs must be bought at pharmacies, diagnostic equipment must be paid for. These and many other of the adjuncts of medical care make difficult, if not impossible, the ancient Samaritanian principle of caring for the poor sick by absorbing the cost—even by giving the innkeeper a denarius and promising to pay more on return. In the face of these institutional changes, how can the noble and generous ethos of medicine respond? Will medicine, like the

Knights Hospitallers, drop the portcullis and draw up the bridge, leaving the unserved without and serving the well insured within?

These are, admittedly, exaggerated images, yet behind the rhetoric lies a real challenge. At a time when the genuine nobility of medicine, a nobility that arises from the science and compassion of men like Sir William Osler, is compromised and threatened from within and without, at a time when many of medicine's younger practitioners either have forgotten or have never learned the ethos of noblesse oblige, the challenge is the choice of an ethos—or rather, the renewed commitment to an ethos. At a certain point in their history, the Knights Hospitallers were faced with a similar choice: they could remain healers of the sick or become rulers and soldiers. They tried to do both, but in the end the ethos of ruling and fighting overwhelmed the ethos of healing. They became builders of fortresses and navies; they amassed a wealth that made them objects of envy to kings and popes. They ended their long history (though they still exist as an honorary and charitable society) as men of power and military might, who eventually fell before the onslaught of still mightier power. The parallel to modern medicine is not too far-fetched. If medicine is to survive as a service, inspired by humane concern, it must choose its ethos and remain faithful to it. The ethos of noblesse oblige, which flows down from power and prestige, is not strong enough to survive the challenge. Sir William, peer of medicine, might well agree.

Our days need a vocabulary and concepts less enmeshed in the ancient and medieval worlds. The traditional ethos of medicine must be invoked from time to time in order to explain the current ethos of medicine, for the present is informed by the past. Still, we must talk about modern problems in more modern terms. Let us move from the ethos of nobility to an ethical doctrine more familiar to the modern ear, the doctrine of rights. The nobility of France renounced its privileges of medieval provenance on August 5, 1789; the Declaration of the Rights of Man was issued by the assembly twenty days later. Our contemporary discourse on ethics hardly remembers the earlier ethos and dwells constantly on the attribution of rights. But the doctrine of rights has a history too, and that history affects how the doctrine applies to the ethics and ethos of medicine.

Chapter 4

Doctor Locke
and Doctors' Rights

An article on the editorial page of the *New York Times* last July was entitled "Meet Dr. Squeezed." The author, Robert Berenson, opened with the comment, "Practicing medicine today means being caught in the middle." Insurers, government agencies, hospitals, one's own patients, put the squeeze on the doctor, as they all press for their own interests or rights. Dr. Berenson continued: "Most doctors accept the inevitable conflicts between cost and quality, patient wishes and clinical judgment, professional autonomy and consumer protection. Nevertheless, physicians feel increasingly beleaguered. Their recommendations and decisions are being questioned, constrained and overruled." [1]

This complaint is a succinct statement of a diffuse problem. Unquestionably the practice of medicine today is vastly more complex than it was only a few years ago. The technology is more elaborate, the institutions are more bureaucratic, the financing is more byzantine. The harassed feeling of the practitioner is the result of many more people, with many more interests, playing a role in what was, not too long ago, a quite simple relationship between a physician and a patient.

Although physicians may *feel* beleaguered, it is really the ethos of medicine that *is* beleaguered. A beleaguered feeling is a psychological phenomenon; it may result from paranoia or from genuine attack. Some persons feel it, some do not. A beleaguered ethos, on the other hand, describes a more objective state of affairs: the values that have long infused a way of life are under attack or, perhaps more accurately, are undermined. A fortress of the Knights of the Hospital could be beleaguered without any of its defenders realizing what was happening: sappers could be digging beneath its foundations. We may say that the ethos of medicine is being sapped.

In the preceding chapter I described an ethos of medicine in terms of nobility. That ethos built upon the duties of the institution of knighthood, stressing the obligation to protect the poor and even inverting the relationship of lord and subject, subordinating the power and interests of the superior to the needs and weakness of the inferior. It is a medieval ethos that reflects the Gospel story of the Good Samaritan. This ethos, gracious and generous as it is, never forgets the position of superiority, and when that position is threatened, it can become defensive. Remnants of this ethos persist within the collective minds and hearts of modern medicine. Noblesse oblige is still the salient ethos, although few modern physicians would think of themselves as nobles. (There are still, however, a few lordly ones among them.)

While it is important to recognize this residue of an ancient ethos, for its presence still influences personal behavior and institutional structures, the description in the antique language of the feudal past may obscure its meaning for moderns.

A contemporary description of the moral relationship between persons might be more comprehensible, especially one that includes the doctrine of rights.

The "squeezed doctor" may react by wondering about his or her "rights." Do not regulatory requirements, institutional restrictions, insurance limitations, malpractice threats, and patient pressures infringe on the right to practice good medicine "according to my ability and judgment," as the Hippocratic oath requires? May not the constraints of a managed-care system inhibit my right to provide the best care for my patients? Is not my right to make a living impaired by proposals to control my income, my choice of a specialty, my place and mode of practice? Are my rights not beleaguered? When the "rights" of one party are squeezed, it is usually the "rights" of some other party that are doing the squeezing.

Some years ago a particularly anguished article in this vein was published—and widely read. Robert Sade proclaimed, "Any physician can say to those who would shackle his judgment and control his profession: I do not recognize your right to my life and my mind, which belong to me and me alone." Dr. Sade defended his proclamation with an argument that seems to appeal to many Americans:

> In a free society, man exercises his right to sustain his own life by producing economic values in the form of goods and services that he is, or should be, free to exchange with other men who are similarly free to trade with him or not. The economic values produced, however, are not given as gifts by nature, but exist only by virtue of the thought and effort of individual men. Goods and services are thus owned as a consequence of

the right to sustain life by one's own physical and mental effort . . . Medical care is neither a right nor a privilege: it is a service that is provided by doctors and others to people who wish to purchase it. It is the provision of his service that a doctor depends upon for his livelihood.[2]

When he wrote these words, Dr. Sade was reacting to certain congressional proposals about health manpower that the president of the American Medical Association at that time called "indentured servitude for physicians." Consequently he stressed the economic rights of physicians. His argument can be generalized to cover the rights of physicians to utilize their skills in accord with their own best judgment in the patient's best interests and to exclude the "third parties" who strive to limit, restrict, control, or dictate the course of clinical care.

Sade's thesis about physicians' rights is derived from an honorable tradition of political philosophy. Although the word and the general notion of "rights" had antecedents in Roman law and medieval political theology, the more modern meaning was formulated in the late Renaissance and came into its own in the seventeenth century. The British philosopher John Locke (1632–1704) was the most eloquent and influential shaper of the modern concept. Locke, known today primarily as a philosopher, was also a physician. He learned and practiced medicine at a time when the ancient art was on the verge of significant changes, and he was the intimate colleague of men who were effecting those changes, particularly Robert Boyle and Thomas Sydenham.[3]

It is somewhat fanciful to connect Locke's philosophy of rights with his experience as a physician, but the fancy may be excused if it sheds some light on the ways in which claims to rights function in the sieges and squeezes of modern medical care. Locke's thinking about rights was compatible with a way of thinking about medicine that he and his friends were generating. That compatibility consisted in being able to think about rights as the exclusive possession of a property and in being able to think about one's medical competence as a property over which one might have dominance. John Locke never said this or anything like it, but the two lines of thought that he entertained, one about politics and one about medicine, can be aligned in a suggestive parallel.

John Locke and Thomas Sydenham were close friends. Locke seems to have served as an amanuensis to Sydenham for several years and certainly learned bedside medicine by going on rounds with the renowned clinician. Sydenham was not an academician or a theoretician; he was a clinician and an empiricist. His contribution to medical science was the initiation of an empirically based nosology in which individual diseases were identified by their discrete signs and symptoms. Quite specific remedies were indicated for each. His clinical descriptions of gout (from which he suffered greatly), dysentery, malaria, measles, smallpox, syphilis, and tuberculosis were masterly. Although honored with the title "the English Hippocrates" because of his emulation of the empirical and naturalist spirit of the Greek, his approach to medicine was radically different. Henry Sigerist explains the difference:

> Hippocrates recognized only disease, not diseases. He knew only sick individuals, only cases of illness. The patient and his

malady were for him inseparably connected as a unique happening, one which would never recur. But what Sydenham saw above all in the patient . . . was the typical, the pathological process which he had observed in others before and expected to see in others again. In every patient there appeared a specific kind of illness. For him, maladies were entities, and his outlook upon illness was, therefore, ontological. Hippocrates wrote the histories of sick persons, but Sydenham wrote the history of diseases.[4]

Sydenham's approach slowly but surely undermined the speculative medical systems, with their univocal and unempirical explanations of disease and its cause, that had dominated the previous centuries. Together with the spirit of scientific investigation into physiology personified by Locke's other friend, Robert Boyle, Sydenham's method created the medical science and art that has persisted to the present time. Diseases are discrete sets of signs and symptoms with discrete pathophysiological causes, which can be explained in general scientific terms. This sort of medicine came into its own, in much more sophisticated form, during the nineteenth century. One significant implication is that a disease, and in principle all diseases, can be dominated and conquered by those who have the skill and the science to recognize and explain them. Physicians become the ones who, in principle, have power over disease.

John Locke lived a diversified life, practicing medicine, expounding philosophy, and engaging in politics. His philosophy mirrored his politics, for he championed civil liberty over royal authority. He was both physician and secretary to the earl of Shaftsbury, a major figure in the cause that in time became the Glorious Revolution. His dedication to this cause cost him his Oxford fellowship and brought him lengthy exile. What he wrote about rights can be understood in the light of these experiences. He was dedicated to creating a social order in which free individuals could claim their own "space" and associate freely with others to share the goods of liberty, knowledge, and enterprise. The political philosopher Ernest Barker describes Locke's philosophy of rights: "There is, Locke taught, a Natural Law rooted and grounded in the reasonable nature of man; there are natural rights to life, liberty, health and property, existing in virtue of such law. Among these, the right of property, in things with which men have mixed their labor, is cardinal." [5]

In addition to explaining and defending the right of property, Locke had a tendency to write about other fundamental rights as if they too were best conceived on the model of property rights: "Man has by nature a power . . . to preserve his property, that is, his life, liberty and estate." Again, "Every man has a property in his own person. This nobody has any right to but himself. The labor of his body and the work of his hands . . . are properly his." [6] Locke maintained that men enter into contracts not only to distribute property among themselves but also to distribute their liberty in certain ways. The state comes into existence because men agree in a social contract to transfer certain of their natural liberties to government. This social contract is also fiduciary, inasmuch as those who transfer liberties to the government entrust the government to act in their best interests.

In two areas the Lockean doctrine has had a definite effect on medical practice and, indirectly, on the thinking of physicians about their role. Both the conferral of special privileges on scientific orthodoxy and the establishment of licensure contribute to the formation of a profession in the modern sense. Its members share an identity, a language, lifetime membership, self-regulation, values, explicit social boundaries, and implicit socialization of new members. Professionals enjoy autonomy based on knowing what is best for the client, subjecting their decisions only to peer review, and establishing standards of behavior through their organization. The autonomy of the medical profession has been ratified in most countries by licensure; the state delegates to the profession, in law and in fact, the authority to educate, admit, and discipline its own members. In turn, the institution of licensure reinforces and defines the profession.

Although the rights of physicians began to be acknowledged in the Middle Ages, when physicians formed guilds and received certain privileges in return for services to the town, the philosophical grounds and the practical conditions for special rights came together only in and after Locke's time. During the past three centuries two conditions have particularly fostered the notion that physicians enjoy special rights. The first has to do with the claim that only those who ascribe to certain systems of medical science should be recognized as physicians and allowed to practice. The second centers on the claim that the activities of physicians create a special relationship between patient and physician over which the physician exercises authority. Both claims assert that the physician should exercise jurisdiction over a range of activities; others are obliged to acknowledge this and are not to interfere.

In the first claim, the range of activities is the teaching and practice of the healing arts; the "others" are those who wish to practice these arts without the requisite orthodox science. In the second claim, the range of activities is the transaction between the physician and the patients who have sought him; the "others" are employers of physicians, contractors of physician services, insurers, and the government. The first claim is justified by an appeal to the value of true knowledge. The second claim is justified by appealing to the benefits that may be bestowed only within the privacy of the relationship. These claims, then, have the structure of a right: assertion of jurisdiction over a sphere of activities, engendering an obligation on certain others to act or refrain from acting in specific ways, and justified by an appeal to a presumably authoritative value. These two historical developments are exemplars of the moral rights of physicians.

During the eighteenth century, in the wake of Sydenham and others, medicine slowly began to become scientific, relying more on evidence than on speculative theory. These developments encouraged orthodoxies that in turn made it possible, many thought, to differentiate scientific from nonscientific practitioners. The orthodox continually proclaimed that the unorthodox, the empirics, the sectarians, and the quacks were harmful. But the strongest claims of orthodoxy depended less upon benefits or the safety of its own medical system than upon its supposed truth, conformity with current science. Legislatures looked with favor upon the medical orthodoxies, and in both England and America legislatures were persuaded to grant licenses and licensing power to associations of practitioners representing, for the most part, the medical orthodoxies.[7]

It soon became apparent that the privileged orthodox were no more or less successful in curing disease than the heterodox. Indeed, some of their methods were seen to be more harmful than those of their competitors. Public skepticism was widespread. It was frequently suggested that the licensure of orthodox medicine created nothing more than a monopoly for the financial benefit of one class of physician. In many jurisdictions licensure laws were repealed or fell into disuse. In the second half of the nineteenth century, however, some impressive demonstrations of efficacy began to appear. The widespread success of inoculation, the results of aseptic surgery, and the therapeutic promise of bacteriology and cellular pathology restored public faith in scientific medicine. Legislatures were persuaded to reenact licensure laws. The argument for licensure was no longer based merely on the possession of a true science but also on the evidence of benefit resulting from the application of that science.

Many of the benefits were readily demonstrable. Yet it was maintained that they could be bestowed only within the context of an interaction in which the physician ordered a regimen and the patient complied. Tuberculosis could be treated by rest and fresh air, infant diarrhea by assiduous sanitation, typhus by strict quarantine. All of these, even though uncomplicated activities, were performed "on doctor's orders." The authority of the physician to dictate the regimen and to see that it was carried out by patients, as well as by those caring for them, was asserted to be an essential condition for realization of the benefits of medicine. Although physician authority and patient compliance have always been integral to the medical transaction, the structure of the transaction was strengthened by the demonstration of benefits.

Another new feature was the belief that the proper relationship between physician and patient could be fostered only within certain social and economic arrangements, which involved rules about consultations, advertising, fee setting, and criticism of colleagues. These arrangements were deemed most suitable for the nurturing of the patient-physician relationship; they centralized authority, created a bond of trust, and encouraged patient compliance. The primary right of the physician was freedom to structure the physician-patient relationship in a way that would yield the benefits his scientific skills enabled him to offer. His title to that right comprised his expertise, his benevolence, and his intention to structure that relationship for the benefit of the patient.[8]

Medical-practice acts devised by the organized profession and passed by legislatures during the second half of the nineteenth century acknowledged this right. Such acts, and all subsequent legislation until quite recently, made no rules that would abrogate the authority of the physician to structure his relationship with the patient. The assumption was that physicians not only were skilled in medical arts but also were benevolent; they had the intention and the motivation to turn medical arts to the benefit of the patient. Skill and benevolence were the titles to the right to control the patient-physician relationship.

within the general rules of free enterprise. Attempts to interfere with the free market by innovations such as prepaid group practice were vigorously rejected by the organized profession. Such innovations, it was claimed, would compromise the discretion of the individual practitioner, encourage in-house consultations, and arouse suspicion that financial considerations would taint both the benevolence and the science of the practitioner. Good medicine—that is, the performance of medical actions based on scientific skills and flowing from benevolence—could be practiced only within the confines of a contract between a patient who freely sought aid and a physician who had full discretion with regard to care. Solo practice, on a fee-for-service basis, was considered to be the optimum social and economic arrangement for such a contract.[10] This is the sort of medicine that John Locke, had he applied his general political philosophy to the work of medicine, might have appreciated. It merits the title "Lockean medicine," and it is the threat to its existence that distresses Robert Sade.

Behind the indignation that many physicians feel at intrusions into their clinical activities may lie a deep conviction that the very essence of being a physician is being challenged. This persuasion might be described in what is, admittedly, a rather whimsical interpretation of Lockean rights. Up to this point, the Lockean claims have concerned the competence one acquires by the study of medicine and the forms of practice that appear to allow one to exercise that competence. My fanciful interpretation goes beyond that: it claims that the physician has a right over the disease itself. Disease, in Sydenham's thinking, became an "entity," a natural thing of a discrete sort in the world and in the body of the patient. Locke considered that "whatsoever a man removes out of the state that nature hath provided and left it in, he hath mixed his labour with it and joined to it something that is his own, and thereby makes it his property." [11] We might speculate that medical skills constitute the labor that the physician mixes with the natural entity of disease and, in so doing, dominates it and makes it his own property. Naturally, this property is dominated only to be destroyed; but still, it belongs in some extended sense to the physician who will master it. An owner of undeveloped land has the right to cut down trees in order to make her property productive. And the physician may destroy disease in order to make the body healthy. In order to do so, he has a right to dominate it: the disease may be in the patient, but it belongs to the physician.

Of course, in order to get at the disease, the physician must go "through" the patient: he needs to gain "right of way." This can be accomplished by contract. Just as Locke viewed the most important human transactions as consensual contracts, the medical transaction is thought of in contractual terms, in which one of the parties hands over certain freedoms in order to obtain the benefits that the other offers. The Lockean-Sydenhamian physician acquires a right over the disease and the patient by double title: he mingles his labor with the disease and masters it; he contracts with the patient to do his work. Even though the physician must get access to the disease through the patient—he cannot trespass—he almost has an independent right over the disease itself.

Perhaps this is too fanciful a conception. Doctors Locke and

Sydenham might laugh at it. Still, it has a ring of veri-similitude: many modern physicians act and talk as if they did have some independent right over a disease. It is a common complaint that physicians are interested only in the disease, not in the patient who has the disease. Is this surprising if the physician believes that he or she has rightful title and claim to the disease itself? The belligerent metaphors of medicine, in which physicians "fight disease with aggressive therapies," suggest that forays into the territory occupied by the enemy may occasionally overrun the rights of the inhabitants. Physicians tend to be indignant if prevented by the patient, or by other interfering bodies, from getting at the site of disease and mastering it. The relatively recent introduction of "informed consent" into the law and ethics of the patient-physician relationship, while a welcome redress of excessive paternalism, still seems to some physicians an affront. They feel that it challenges unduly their commitment to the patient's welfare. Some few physicians find the patient's right to refuse medical ministration to be more than an affront; to them it is an outrage.

The feeling of being beleaguered arises when one's property is invaded, when one's rights are infringed. The many invasions felt by physicians come from patients' claims over their bodies and minds—which, in the Lockean metaphor, belong to the physician, at least when those bodies and minds are diseased. Invasions also come from regulators, insurers, lawyers, and others who erect barriers between physicians and the sphere of work that is rightly their property. Again, these are exaggerated images, but they make explicit the attitudes that seem to lie beneath the surface.

During the last century, then, physicians have built around themselves fortresses of rights. This is an understandable reaction of embattled nobility. Even with willingness to serve and dedication to service, protection of territory and privilege can become a dominant concern. One commentator on John Locke's philosophy described it as "possessive individualism": each person is a nobleman in his own castle. His rights are constituted by the walls that keep others out and by the ability to extend (by honest means) the boundaries of his safe demesne.[12] This thesis was, of course, an appropriate reaction to the claims of omnipotence uttered by monarchs who ruled, they claimed, "by divine right." It is not quite an appropriate concept for the work of physicians.

The rights of physicians over their practices, over the disease, and even over their patients were bound to be challenged. The era of Lockean rights in medical practice came to an end in Locke's own England in 1946 with the enactment of the National Health Service Law, and it began to recede in the United States with the passage of Medicare and Medicaid in 1965. Here the organized profession had, since the 1920s, opposed compulsory health insurance in the name of the physician-patient relationship. That argument was eventually refuted by the rejoinder that the relationship simply did not exist for millions of Americans whose poverty denied them access to "mainstream medicine," that is, to fee-for-service medical care. The American remedy for this situation was fashioned in a way which, if not Lockean in substance, was so in spirit. It left the "property rights" of physicians intact and undertook to pay the physicians on a fee-for-service basis out of an insurance fund or public monies. The legislation affirmed that there was no intent to change in any way the practice of medicine.[13] Lockean medicine seemed safe, but that safety was spurious.

In the thirty years since that promise, it has become evident that federal payment for medical services has changed medical practice in major ways. The government has an interest in controlling costs; accordingly, it limits reimbursement and reviews quality of care. It encourages prepayment group practice in the belief that this is a more efficient and economical form for delivery of services. In addition to the regulations generated by federal involvement in health care, threats to the authority of physicians arise on other frontiers. These are extensions of legal restraints into areas in which physicians previously had exercised personal discretion: the changing technological context of medical practice and the growing perception of a "right to health care." Each of these raises questions about certain settled rights of the medical profession and poses against them emerging rights of other parties.

The benevolent skill that gave Lockean title to the professionals' claim over their practices, over disease, and even over their patients has in recent years been the object of some skepticism. The term "paternalism" has been applied, suggesting that even when benevolent, the skill has been used in the authoritarian manner of parent toward ignorant and wayward child. (Those who worry about paternalism would be edified by Locke's wonderful essay, *Thoughts Concerning Education*.) Patients have been infantalized by physicians, who derogated to themselves the discretion patients have a right to exercise over their own bodies and lives. Granted that patients do not know as much medicine as their doctors, patients know as much and more about their own values and interests. In the 1970s a good deal of criticism was directed against medical paternalism, and patient autonomy became the central concept of the nascent "bioethics."

Paternalism may be criticized on other grounds. The title of benevolent skill rested on the notion that, like Locke's natural man, the physician "mixed his labor," a combination of skills and benevolence, into a human transaction producing a peculiar property, the patient-physician relationship. Today, however, we see that this human transaction has become more complex (even as industrialism rendered Locke's simple notion of property problematic). Many other hands mix their labor to make the medical transaction possible. The patient's active role in the transaction makes the so-called contract appear somewhat less "fiduciary" than in the past. Determinants of disease and health that fall outside the range of medical intervention call for skills other than medical. Finally, economists have helped us to recognize that it is not the patients, seeking the care of doctors, who determine the volume of care given. It is rather the doctors, by selecting those in need of treatment, prescribing medication, recommending surgery, and ordering admittance to hospitals, who create the volume, and to a great extent the cost, of medical care. The power to prescribe is a great power.

It is easy to see that this power may serve self-interest rather than benevolence. In Medicaid scandals, medically questionable procedures were ordered by physicians for their own profit. "Managed care" makes it possible to skimp on medically indicated procedures to improve the plan's bottom line. Such practices, while hardly prevalent, cast a shadow over benevolent intent and dim the trust that should bind patient and physician. It is no longer plausible to consider medical skill as a kind of property which, in Sade's words, the physician is "free to exchange with other men who are free to trade with him or not." [14]

Challenges to the benevolent authority of physicians also arise from the changing technological and scientific capacities of medicine. New diagnostic procedures uncover disease prenatally or disclose diseases that previously ran a hidden course until irreparable damage had been done. Resuscitative techniques can revive premature newborns or the seriously traumatized, who formerly would have died but now may continue to survive in a damaged state. Supportive measures sustain comatose patients and the dying, for whom no therapeutic measures are available.

These technological advances have aroused public concern about the appropriateness of leaving to the physician the crucial choices inherent in their use. Do not the issues here go far beyond medical skill and into public policy? Should physicians be allowed to make a prenatal diagnosis that may lead to abortion of a fetus merely because it is male or female? Should genetic screening, which may mislead, confuse, or socially compromise individuals or groups, be placed in the hands of physicians? Should premature babies be saved if their future lives hold little promise? Should an abortus born alive be resuscitated? Should physicians be allowed to terminate artificially supported life? With regard to all this technology, are the costs justified by the outcome? Physicians determine the use of expensive diagnostic and therapeutic technology: is this fair to the patients, to their families, or to society? These questions cast doubt on the propriety of the physician as a decision maker about the technology that has become an intrinsic part of medical practice. Indeed, many critics of modern medicine proclaim that physicians, armed with technology, create more ills than they cure.

These questions reflect doubt not about physicians' skills but about their benevolence. That important title to physician rights is clouded because it is felt that even the best-intentioned and most selfless physicians are not in a position to perceive or control the "best interests" of others. Their judgment must be supplemented and supplanted by that of others. In many cases the "other" is the government. So the medical profession, beneficiary of Lockean rights for several centuries, now finds itself face to face with the Lockean rights of others. Like John Locke himself, who in his political and philosophical life struggled to apportion rights of life, liberty, and property among monarchy, government, and citizens, modern medicine must find the proper apportionment of rights among its own practitioners, its patients, and those who pay for their services, the government and the citizenry.

Locke, while a proponent of individual rights, was also a proponent of a civil society in which free individuals could live cooperatively and peacefully. More than any other philosopher, he laid the intellectual groundwork for the institutions of democratic government. In the social contract he proposed that autonomous individuals grant powers to a government that will assure them freedom in the development of their property and in the pursuit of their beliefs. Again, in the new situation of modern medicine, Lockean philosophy provides a model: the autonomous physician contracts with the autonomous patient to create a democracy of medicine. In today's world the Lockean physician's contract with the patient is much more than the granting of a right-of-way through the patient to the disease; it is a compact that sets out the assumptions, conditions, and sanctions contingent on the entering of the relationship. The legal and ethical concept of "informed consent" encapsulates the new, expanded contract.

In this contract the old "noble" justification for paternalism is banished. The basis for the "therapeutic privilege," whereby a physician justified withholding distressing information from a patient, is demolished. Therapeutic privilege depends on the perception of a radical inequality between patient and physician. In the democracy of present-day medicine this inequality is abolished by proclamation of the rights of patients, who now come to physicians as equal partners in care.

This commendable ideal carries the Lockean view of human relations to its logical conclusion: from the possessive individualism of physicians as proprietors of their skills to the cooperative, contractual relationship between autonomous physicians and autonomous patients. The master and the serf have become equals. Like all democracies, though, this one is fragile. Claimed equality does not ever correspond to actual equality of power, resources, possessions, and self-image. In every democracy radical inequalities continue to exist. The problem of justice in a democracy is the continual, incremental equalizing of inequalities. In the democracy of medicine the inequalities are many: social prestige, knowledge, training, and the possession of technology on the physician's side, physical and psychological disability, financial burdens, and unfamiliarity with the health-care world on the other. The free and equal democracy of medicine that ethics and law envision may be more an ideal than an actuality. Certainly, its ideal conditions are neglected and circumvented more frequently than would be tolerated in a true political democracy. The ideal of "informed consent," for example, is pocked with peculiar exceptions: "implied consent," "substituted consent," and, perhaps most frequently, "alienated consent"—in which the patient simply "lets the doctor decide." Similarly, the modern problem of malpractice vitiates the social contract between patients and physicians. To be sure, the existence of the law to enforce contractual arrangement is an essential of the social contract. But when the parties to the contract get into the habit of going to the law rather than engaging in conciliation and negotiation, the free contract appears increasingly coercive. The tradition of Lockean rights in medicine prevails, but in a fragile and imperfect democracy.

Lockean medical rights must be melded with the earlier traditions of medical duty reviewed in previous chapters. Even if a case can be made that physicians have a property right in their competence and license to practice, this right cannot provide an exclusive description of the ethos and ethics of medicine. If medicine is conceived in this way, most of the traditional ethics is forgotten and with it much of medicine's

Chapter 5

Bentham in His Box

Englishmen are known for their eccentricities. Consider this funeral service: The corpse of Jeremy Bentham, one of England's most respected and influential men, lay on a dissecting table at the Webb Street School of Anatomy in London. His personal physician, Southwood Smith, delivered the eulogy before a select group of Bentham's friends and disciples—then, without further ceremony, dissected the cadaver. Dr. Smith was acting on instructions in Bentham's will, directing that his body be used for anatomical dissection "so that mankind may reap some small benefit by my disease."[1] The eulogist-dissector had expounded on this bequest, noting that it represented a poignant example of the deceased's fundamental philosophical principle of utility, the promotion of the greatest happiness to the greatest number. Happiness, Smith stated, depended on health; health depended on medical care, which depended on medical science, which depended on dissection. Ergo, bodies should be dissected.

That unconventional funeral took place on June 9, 1832. The great man had died three days before, after eighty-four productive, happy, healthy years. Bentham, however, is still in our midst. He, or rather his mummy, sits in a glass box in University College, London. He had decided that an "auto-icon" would bring some pleasure to future generations, who might wonder what so famous a man looked like. Wearing his best straw hat, hand resting on "Dapple" (his favorite walking stick), he gazes benignly at the dons, students, and curious visitors. He even was trundled out to attend a sherry on the occasion of the founding of the Bentham Society. The *New York Times* reported, "The auto-icon, which bears a resemblance to the comedian Jack Benny, looked distantly pleased." [2]

Jeremy Bentham does not enter our story of *The New Medicine and the Old Ethics* because of his contribution to the new medicine. He was by profession a lawyer, by avocation a social philosopher and reformer. His fertile mind inquired everywhere and "invented" (a preferred word of his) schemes and plans for the improvement of mankind's lot in every department. Primarily interested in the reform of law and government, he advised rulers and politicians in his own land and throughout Europe (he was an honorary citizen of France). Although he wrote little about medicine and health, two of his disciples, Southwood Smith and Edwin Chadwick, were inspired by his schemes of social reform and applied them to problems of public health. Chadwick, who was Bentham's amanuensis for a time, presided over the first major public health reforms in modern times and in 1842 produced the monumental and influential *Report on the Sanitary Condition of the Labouring Population of Great Britain*. He championed the installation of ceramic-pipe sewers, flushed with running water to banish human wastes from the fetid cities to distant depositories. Dr. John Snow's famous denunciation of the

Broad Street pump as the source of cholera would have come to little had not the plan of what one author calls "the arterio-venous system of water supply and sewage disposal" been implemented in London and in most of the major cities of Europe and America.[3]

Bentham, then, in his character of social reformer did inspire a significant contribution to public health. He also proposed the establishment in the cabinet of a Ministry of Health that was to oversee the water supply, supervise conditions in factories, and suppress harmful drugs—a suggestion that was implemented in Great Britain only in 1919 and in the United States in 1953. Bentham, however, appears in our pages less as a contributor to the new medicine and more as the presiding genius of a new ethic that is achieving some popularity in the new medicine. Bentham is sometimes called the father of utilitarianism, although credit for the utilitarian "principle of the greatest happiness" probably belongs elsewhere and although he himself paid little attention to the elaboration of a philosophical system. Nevertheless, he earns the title because of his insistent promotion of the idea that social reform in law, suffrage, criminal justice, economics, education, and many other areas of life should promote the "greater good," and that the greater good consisted in maximizing pleasure over pain. But more than the promotion of principle makes Bentham important for the modern world. He realized that the promotion of principle required rigorous analysis of facts, and systematic application of that analysis to institutional programs and structures. Principles were always to be aimed at practice. This was in his time a new ethic;

Bentham and his colleagues were called the "radical philosophers." While utilitarianism is no longer a "new ethic," it is appearing as a new message in medicine and health care.

The new medicine hears Bentham's ghostly voice urging all physicians to convert to utilitarianism. Many will not understand the message. Some do not know what utilitarianism is; others may think they have always been utilitarians. Still others may wonder why the voice is urging conversion now. Those who do not understand utilitarianism can be sent to the books. There they will find that it names a philosophical system of ethics that goes far beyond enunciation of the "greatest happiness" principle. Bentham was himself rather casual about the meaning and logical implications of the principle: he was eager to see it put to use in social reform. His secular godchild, John Stuart Mill, elaborated the philosophy in more detail and the Cambridge philosopher Henry Sidgwick expounded on it at great length. Ever since, distinguished philosophical minds have spelled out the implications of the principle of utility in an intricate set of words and concepts, trying to make the system perfectly logical and impregnable to criticism. Others, just as distinguished, have attacked it ruthlessly and, to their satisfaction, demolished its logic. The ideas that seemed so obvious to Bentham, namely, that the springs of all human action are the seeking of pleasure and the avoidance of pain, and that all human activity aims to maximize pleasure over pain, are now entwined in a tangle of explanation, qualification, justification, and criticism.[4]

The physician who goes to the books, then, might find them daunting. Nonetheless, he will begin to see why Mr.

Bentham's ghostly whisper urges conversion to utilitarianism. That doctrine promises some resolution to the pressing problem of allocation of scarce health-care resources that we reflected upon in our parable of the Good Samaritan. Some philosophers have suggested that the principle of utility is particularly appropriate for this problem: one of the earliest commentators on Dr. Scribner's dilemma concerning selection of patients for hemodialysis justifies the use of a criterion of future contribution by noting that "moral philosophers of the present day are pretty well in consensus that the justification of human action is to be sought largely and primarily—if not exclusively—in the principles of utility and justice."[5] As our inquiring physician reads further, he or she might wonder whether the utilitarian principle can be reconciled with a doctor's work. One philosopher points this out cogently:

Suppose that I, a simple Utilitarian, entrust the care of my health to a simple Utilitarian doctor. Now I know that his intentions are generally beneficent towards me. Thus, while he will not malevolently kill me off, I cannot be sure that he will always try to cure me of my afflictions; I can be sure only that he will do so, unless his assessment of the general happiness leads him to do otherwise . . . I could not get him to promise, in the style of the Hippocratic Oath, always and only to deploy his skills to my advantage . . . He would of course keep this promise only if he judged it best on the whole to do so; knowing that, I could not unquestioningly rely on his keeping it; and knowing that, he would realize that, since I would not do so, it would matter that much less if he did keep it. And so on, until his "promise" becomes perfectly idle . . . If general felicific beneficence were the only criterion, then promising and talking alike would become wholly idle pursuits.[6]

This little morality play between the simple utilitarian patient and the simple utilitarian doctor may not please academic utilitarians: they will say it oversimplifies their complex doctrine. Still, it may give pause to patient and physician alike, for they probably enter into their relationship intending and expecting that the doctor must look to the patient's needs, not to the general welfare. Suppose that, as they read in the books of the utilitarian philosophers, they encounter this argument, made by Peter Singer, a brilliant contemporary follower of Bentham. Singer proposes that defective children can be killed. Using as an example a child with hemophilia, he argues:

> When the death of a defective infant will lead to the birth of another infant with better prospects for a happy life, the total amount of happiness will be greater if the defective infant is killed. The loss of a happy life for the first infant is outweighed by the gain of a happier life for the second. Therefore, if killing the hemophiliac infant has no adverse effect on others it would . . . be right to kill him.[7]

The hematologist caring for the child in question would very probably be appalled at Singer's suggestion. The philosopher might respond that the doctor should become a simple utilitarian. Once he saw the system as a whole, he would recognize the cogency of the argument. But conversion to this strange doctrine is not easy for doctors. Even though they may be deeply committed to the general welfare and work intently for the public health, they have been inculcated into the old ethics, which tell them their primary duty must be to their patients. Killing them for the sake of other not yet existing persons seems incredible. Yet the philosopher will retort that, incredible though it seems, it is rational. His ethics is an eminently rational system, logically moving from a simple, irrefutable first principle to particular, practical decisions.

I will not insist that the doctor I have sent to the library remain there too long. Reading the abundant debates over the validity and the interpretation of utilitarianism would absorb many more hours than the average physician could spare. The apparent incompatibility between dedication to one's patient and maximization of the greater good may even be open to resolution. Some competent medical ethicists are convinced utilitarians and believe that the doctrine does not undermine patient care; indeed, many medical ethicists, whatever their doctrinal flavor, admit to the cogency of the utilitarian position for some problems, such as the allocation of scarce resources. I have not rolled out Jeremy Bentham's auto-icon to resuscitate the debate over utilitarianism as a philosophy or its application to medical ethics. I invoke his memory for another purpose, namely, to reflect on the way in which his characteristic rationality has affected medicine and health care.

The utilitarians, under Bentham's tutelage, produced a new set of ethics in the early nineteenth century. It was radical in many features, among which one has had a pervasive effect on modern culture. Bentham loved systems. His characteristic rationality was the "invention" of well-ordered schemes of ideas that could be translated into well-arranged schemes of action. He spoke of a "logic of the will," whereby clearly defined concepts, resulting from analyses of factual states of affairs, were translated into effective solutions of social problems. In an era when government functioned with little information about the condition of public affairs and when "policy" referred more to the secret schemes of rulers and their ministers than to informed, planned interventions, Bentham continually urged rationally constructed social planning based on facts. He was frustrated, when attempting to reform the Poor Laws, to find that no official knew how many poor there were in England. He wrote, "Address yourself to those who feed the hungry—feed them in mass—ask them how many mouths there are to feed—chuck (i.e. plenty) is still the answer." [8]

The spirit of Bentham is incarnate in modern technology. He prided himself on being an inventor. Although he used the word "inventor" in its classic sense of one who discovers the ideas and expression appropriate to the solution of a problem, he would have appreciated it in its later sense of a maker of ingenious machines. Bentham would have enjoyed meeting Thomas Edison. The Englishman lived at the height of the Industrial Revolution and manifested its spirit in his thought: he wanted to make things work. He wanted to make government, economics, and education work to produce the greatest happiness for the greatest number. He was, in a sense, a technologist of the public good.

Throughout his life Bentham was fascinated by the Panopticon, a planned building with a central control tower from which would radiate the spokes for whatever activity the building was used. (It was actually Jeremy's brother Sam who had come up with the idea.) Although Jeremy tried unsuccessfully to promote the Panopticon as a model for English prisons, he could see its utility also for factories, schools, poorhouses, even for a national network of workshops of industry.

Bentham would be delighted with contemporary intensive-care units, for they are his Panopticon realized. Their design would please him and the technology would intrigue him. He would be impressed by the way in which these modern Panopticons integrate machines and personal work into efficient units. Once he realized that this amount of effort produced so little restored health and renewed happiness, his enthusiasm might wane, but he would certainly appreciate the principle of this technology for the efficient delivery of critical care.

Now we can see why Bentham should be present at a discussion of the new medicine. He was a technological thinker, and the new medicine is above all technological. If there is anything that makes a new ethic necessary in the new medicine, it is the dominance of technology. We frequently hear the truism "Medical ethics are changing because of the incredible technological advances in medicine." A closer examination of that commonplace may be worthwhile.

I should clarify my use of the word "technology." I do not mean machines, or the use of machines, or even the network of machinery and its users (although I shall return to these features of technology). I look to the etymology of the word, namely, "an understanding *(logos)* of making or producing *(techne)*. Technology, as I use the word, refers to the ways in which we characteristically *think* of production, that is, how we think through the steps of bringing about some result and order those steps in a patterned sequence so as to be able to repeat them. This sort of thinking is, as Mr. Bentham appreciated, very close to action and production. Thus, technology in its more familiar sense comes into being. It describes the apparatus built to perform the systematic steps; the techniques, or patterned logic and skills, needed to produce and use the apparatus and to interpret its work; and, finally, the organization of people required to run the apparatus and make use of its products.

Behind the apparatus, techniques, and organization is the fundamental attribute of technology: a rational system for replicating results. Authors who reflect on the nature of technology consistently call attention to this feature. The sociologist Daniel Bell writes, "Technology is not simply a machine but a systematic, disciplined approach to objectives, using a calculus of precision and measurements and a concept of systems."[9] Victor Ferkiss, a political scientist, offers a similar, more expansive definition: "Technology is a self-conscious organized means of affecting the physical or social environment, capable of being objectified and transmitted to others, and effective largely independently of the subjective dispositions and personal talents of those involved."[10]

In each of these definitions the systematic, methodical realization of objectives is stressed. In light of this, technology in medicine refers to a complex of medical thinking, medical devices, and coordination of medical workers. It is the logic of diagnosis and therapy, and the application of skills and maneuvers, that might be called technique. It is the employment of manufactured products, such as devices for diagnosis and therapy as well as drugs, that can be called the apparatus of medicine. All this is, I believe, Benthamite thinking. The man who wanted, more than anything else, to make things work would be delighted at the evolution of medicine from random intervention to rational technology. Still, the triumph of technology in medicine creates some difficulties that, for lack of a better term, we describe as ethical problems.

Once it is clear that we are talking, not just about apparatus, but about techniques, apparatus, and organization, we can begin to glimpse the nature of those problems. Technology involves systematic thinking and acting to produce results in a reliable manner. That systematic thinking, in our time, takes the form of statistical reasoning, the technique of counting events in accord with rules for drawing conclusions of a stated level of reliability, Bentham, often frustrated by the total absence of data needed to pursue his reform projects, encouraged the new science of statistics. In fact, several years before his death he was a founder of the Statistics Society. His disciples in the sanitary reform movement, Smith and Chadwick, transformed previously primitive methods of collecting mortality and morbidity data into useful instruments of social policy.

Statistics has become indispensable, not only in public health but in clinical medicine. Ever since the 1830s, when the French physician Pierre Louis devised his "numerical method" of determining the efficacy of a procedure (he was the first to show that bleeding was useless for almost all medical conditions), medicine has become increasingly statistical. The science of epidemiology—the study of the incidence, prevalence, and periodicity of disease—was pioneered in the mid-nineteenth century by Dr. William Farr, who though not a disciple of Bentham was a leader in the sanitary movement that Bentham so deeply influenced. Because of that movement, "it was mainly in London that the science of Medical Statistics had its brilliant origin and early development." [11]

The introduction in the 1930s by Sir A. Bradford Hill and Sir Roland Fischer of sound statistical methods for controlled trials made it imperative that safety and efficacy be determined statistically rather than by personal intuition or experience. In recent years epidemiology and the science of clinical trials have turned to the evaluation of various therapies and the outcomes of various diseases, treated or untreated. Efforts have been made to predict the probabilities of success or failure of interventions for patients with certain conditions. Studies of patients admitted to intensive-care units with varying degrees and combinations of pathological conditions attempt to show what their chance of survival will be. Patients treated for cancer or undergoing major cardiac surgery are placed in categories to which percentages can be attached. In disease after disease and for treatment after treatment, statistical information is increasingly available. Medical journals are filled with statistics; the newspapers herald a relatively modest, but statistically significant improvement in a therapy as a "miracle cure." One wonders whether either the journal readers or the newspaper perusers comprehend the numbers.

Still, this mode of thinking, sharpened to a high degree of

sophistication, is indisputably valuable for medicine. At the same time it reveals the first ethical problem of technological medicine. The patient is an individual. Every practitioner knows that a patient with a 10 percent chance of survival can fall either in the 90 percent or the 10 percent category, that even when diagnostic studies reveal a 90 percent chance that no disease is present there is a 10 percent chance of lethal cancer. Even though the language of statistics is spoken (often in a broken dialect) in every clinic and ward, practitioners recognize that the patient being assigned to this or that statistical category is really a "statistic of one."

Physicians are heirs to an ethic that requires dedication to individual patients. They seriously accept the welfare of patients as their primary—indeed, sometimes their sole—responsibility. And patients rightly expect this of their physicians. Yet, as physicians think through diagnosis and devise therapy, they do so technologically. This is, of course, an enormous benefit to the patients: their treatment is not based on the random experience and untested intuition of their doctor. At the same time, the certitude of statistical thinking is limited: decisions based on that thinking depend in actuality on a profoundly moral factor: the risk of being wrong that any physician is willing to tolerate. Some physicians sanction little risk; they repudiate the statistical in favor of a "do everything" attack. They are the physicians who will always take the last-ditch stand, who see no case as hopeless, who will pursue every diagnostic clue regardless of cost. Other physicians accept more risk, hew close to the statistical norm and, in so doing, may appear cold and careless of the individual patient. Physicians of neither type are "unethical." They merely highlight the first ethical problem with medical technology, namely, the gap between statistical thinking and dedication to individual well-being.

The second problem appears when we note that technology provides a multiplicity of readily applied techniques. The techniques are ready-made and at hand: they do not have to be laboriously compounded or constructed on each occasion. Stethoscope and sphygmomanometer, CT scanner and dialyzer, penicillin and diazepam all exist and are ready to use. They are products of the twentieth century. The pharmacopoeia of Bentham's Dr. Smith had to be compounded by hand. Yet illness runs a capricious course and, as every physician knows, the value of intervention varies at different points in that course. In many cases the available techniques are enormously beneficial: an electrocardiogram can dispel fear of serious cardiac arrhythmia; dopamine can quickly reverse plummeting blood pressure. Still, ready techniques can attract precipitous action. Intervention before the diagnostic picture is clear can be disastrous or can unnecessarily lead to a long, hard course. Iatrogenic harm, caused by the treatment itself, results in part from this precipitous approach. Thus, one able clinician is said to have admonished his residents, "Don't do something, just stand there!" In order to be rightly applied, technology must be timely applied. It may be that the technological armamentarium has obscured one of the essential features of medical ethics: the ability to wait and see. At the same time, it may have dampened interest in chronic disease, about which "little or nothing" can be done: little or nothing being defined in relation not to the patient's need but to the absence of a condition against which the available technologies can be mobilized.

A third problem appears when we note that technology aims at reliably produced results. A successful technology is one that is applied in the assurance that the objective will be met. The results are produced "like clockwork" (the earliest of the modern technologies has left its imprint on the language). Antibiotics almost invariably will clear up infections caused by identified organisms; if they fail, one suspects that the organism has become resistant or was improperly identified. The ventilator will sustain respiration infallibly unless there is a concomitant problem such as airway resistance or massive loss of lung tissue.

Although these reliable results are the products of technology, they may not always benefit the patient. Reaching the goal of a technology is a "good." Aristotle pointed out long ago that the primary meaning of "good" is the fulfillment of a goal, but the goal may not be a good in the life of the one who is affected. The cure of pneumonia in a very old, demented person with cancer is a dubious benefit; artificially maintained respiration of an irreversibly comatose person is a doubtful good. Evaluation of a result as a benefit requires a much more complex, more personal, and more humane consideration than recognition of the result itself. It may be that the high reliability and replicability of results that technology makes possible obscure the difference between a result and a benefit. Doing "everything" is ambiguous when we do not know whether this is a promise to produce every possible result or an assurance that only the beneficial results will be pursued.

Finally, technology requires an organization of persons.

Many individuals, with varying skills, must cooperate to create and apply techniques. The requisite organization may range from a loose association of scholars and scientists in a particular field to a tightly knit clinical team. Each participant understands a facet of the complex structure and will focus expert attention on that facet. When decisions are made about patients, however, the many minds of the technological organization must focus on the patient. Clearly, the attending physician will make decisions, but the other participants must contribute their professional opinions and, at the very least, be aware of the reasons behind the final decisions. In the process, the organization must coalesce into a community—it must move from being disparate parts of the technology to participants in its rational use. This goal is not easy to accomplish; divergence of opinion and differences in view often lead to confusion, even conflict. The patient will inevitably suffer.

We sometimes speak of the "interface" between technology and medicine; that is, the way in which machines and techniques fit, or do not fit, into the activities of caring and curing. We have noted at least four problems at that interface: the disparity between statistical thinking and personal dedication, the temptation to precipitous action, the confusion between results and benefits, and the potential for conflict in organization. There are more obstacles, but enough has been said to show that the word "interface" is misleading: in fact, no interface may be possible. In its original meaning, taken from electronics, "interface" refers to the way in which one electronic system contacts and energizes another. Thus, applied to technology and medicine, this term implies that somehow the values of personal dedication, cautious waiting, determination to benefit, and community will flow into systematic thinking, ready availability of technique, and reliability of results. Thereby these values will somehow "energize" technology with humanity.

I suspect that this is the wrong image to describe the relationship. Technology is what it is and should remain what it is. It is a human achievement of extraordinary ingenuity and utility that is quite distinct from the human accomplishment of ethical values.

Jeremy Bentham serves as a symbol of this separation between the technology of medicine and the ethics of medicine. We return to him, not now recalling his productive life and fertile mind, but viewing his present state as an immobile auto-icon encased in a box. His waxen face fronts on the world "distantly pleased"—distantly, because behind the waxen face there is no vital mind, heart, or voice to engage us and draw us into conversation. Boxed in, Bentham can no longer reach out to touch the world of government, law, economics, and social intercourse that he affected during his life. This is, in a way, a symbol of the distance between technology and ethics. The systematic efficacy of technology does not reach infallibly to persons. It reaches systematically toward general happiness and must be pulled toward individuals by the quite personal decisions we call ethical.

How can this be done? First of all, we must admit that in modern medical and scientific education, there is very little teaching about technology. There is plenty of teaching *of* technology—how to create it, apply it, evaluate it—but as for teaching *about* the meaning of technology—its impact on human life and institutions, its overt and covert effects on many practices—very little is taught. This is particularly true in medical education, where techniques dominate the philosophy of technique almost to the point of extinguishing it. The medical student or graduate physician learns much about the technologies of medical care and the science that underlies their use, but learns next to nothing about how those techniques are modifying the meaning and the ethics of medicine and of the patient-physician relationship.

There is a distance between technological thinking and ethical thinking. But technology and ethics are not foreigners, they are neighbors in the world of human accomplishment. They face each other, rather than interface. The personal face of ethics looks at the impersonal face of technology in order to comprehend technology's potential and its limits; the face of technology looks to ethics in order to be directed to human purposes and benefits. This "*intra*facing" will be often critical and sometimes conflicting. Both ethics and technology should profit from the inspection: ethics by becoming more appreciative of the possibilities for human benefit opened up by systems, technology by becoming more amenable to the need for humane evaluation of its methods and products.

Asklepios' reptile was a healing creature: in ancient mythology the snake, whose skin was shed and rejuvenated, symbolized eternity and restoration of life and health. The temples of Asklepios were infested with snakes, said to be *Coluber longissima*, a large but quite harmless creature. In the porches of these Asklepeona the sleeping sick dreamed that they were approached by serpents who healed them by a touch of their tongue. That healing tongue becomes in the *Time* cover the forked tongue of a venomous reptile. Shocking as the picture is to those who believe in the beneficence of medicine, it draws on a deeper meaning of the symbol of the snake. One commentator of the rod and staff of Asklepios speaks of "the ancient conception of the serpent as the embodiment of the mystery of the one absolute life of the earth, which entails a continual dying and resurrection . . . the combination of corruption and salvation, of darkness and light, of good and evil in the Asklepian symbol."[2] Another writes, "These animals symbolize life at the threshold of death, a hidden force, dark and cold, but at the same time, warm and radiant, that stirs beneath the surface of the waking world and accomplishes the miracle of cure."[3] The snake is fearsome and fascinating.

The true symbolism of the snake in medicine consists not in the superficial image of the doctor as "snake in the grass," but in the deeper ambiguity of the power of sickness and the power of healing. The history of medicine reveals this ambiguity again and again. Illness is a time of crisis, a dividing point between comfort, capability, and life on the one hand, and pain, loss, and death on the other. The physician claims to be able to guide the patient through that crisis by knowledge and skill. But even the guidance itself is dangerous, for knowledge is fallible and skill can slip. With this in mind, the Hippocratic writers remind physicians that "interventions are perilous" and that "when the disease grows strong, in the perplexity of the moment, most things are likely to go wrong."[4] Both illness and medicine are ambiguous. It is possible to speculate that the problem of medical ethics is, at root, the problem of living and working within that ambiguity. When the Hippocratic physician swore to "act for the benefit of my patient . . . and do no harm or injustice," he expressed the ambiguity of his art, capable of wounding physically and harming morally, and at the same time "bringing relief from pain and the mitigation of the power of disease."[5] The "good" physician must recognize this ambiguity and intently incline toward the good side. This is the oldest feature of the old ethics of medicine.

We have reviewed the phases of those old ethics from their origin in Hippocratic medicine to contemporary times, proposing that their earliest phase stressed the imperatives of competence, in the pursuit of benefit and avoidance of harm for one's patients; that the second phase promoted compassion and generous self-sacrifice in the care of the sick; that the third phase envisioned the nobility of service; and that the final and most recent phase initiated a kind of democracy of medicine. Each of these phases continues into the subsequent ones in definite but subtle ways. At the same time, we have seen the growth of medicine's technical knowledge and power as it becomes, in the words of the *Time* article, "ever more precise." We have noted that even as it becomes more precise, it faces problems never encountered by the competent, compassionate, and dedicated physicians of the past. They never had to ask Who is the patient? They never were aware of the unending line of people seeking help. They never worked within institutional or financial structures and strictures as complex as their modern counterparts. The question that has been posed again and again in the previous pages is whether the old ethics can inform the new medicine in ways that mitigate the ambiguities that even ancient physicians saw in their work.

Where is the mix of myth and modern medicine taking us? How does reflection on the old ethics, with their antique images and language, help us to manage the ambiguities? Are we not better off discarding the myths? Must we not formulate new ethics to fit the new medicine? I think not. Instead, we must revive the meaning of the old ethics and bring that refreshed meaning to the new problems. And the old ethics to be revived are not one strand alone, the Hippocratic-Cabotean or the Samaritanian or the noble dedication to service, but all of these woven together. This is the new cloth woven out of old threads.

The first problem posed by the new medicine facing the old ethics was the limits of competence. The Hippocratic ethic enjoined competence and restraint; the Cabotean ethic specified competence as the mastery of diagnostics and therapeutics, requiring that the "benefits" and "harms" of the ancient injunction be translated into specific clinical effects for the presenting patient. The new medicine, based on molecular genetics and capable of organ, cell, and gene transplantation, blurs the image of the presenting patient. Populations of potential patients now appear behind the presenting patient. The question posed to the ethics of competence is, To whom and when should the powers of medicine be administered? What are the moral limits of competence? Thus, we chose Dr. Scribner and his first chronic-dialysis patient, Clyde Shields, as the pioneers of the new medicine: the technique used to save Shields from imminent death became, first, a paradigm of too many patients waiting for treatment, then a paradigm of too many patients being treated. Behind Clyde Shields stood crowds of the untreated and clusters of the overtreated. The question was insistently asked, Who should be dialyzed and when?

The ancient ambiguity appears in another form: Must we snatch some from death when we know others will be left to die? Must we snatch from death when we suspect that the saved life will differ radically in quality from its prior state? The ethics of competence alone are inadequate to answer those questions. Compassion must supplement competence. Recall that the Good Samaritan parable concludes with the cate-chism: "Which now of these three . . . was neighbor unto him that fell among the thieves? And he said, He that shewed mercy on him. Then said Jesus unto him, Go, and do thou likewise."

The key word for the renewed ethics of medicine is "neigh-bor," that is, one with whom one can converse, for whom one can do favors, and from whom one can expect help in turn. Compassion looks at the restoration of vital living and human intercourse. It is a parody of compassion to revive and preserve life without human activity. One of the ethical limits of competence is compassionless efficacy, the application of technologies that have low probabilities of restoring an active life. This blending of competence and compassion provides a rule for all intensive care: intervene only as long as it is reasonable to expect a return to human intercourse. The object of care is to restore not a life but a neighbor.

Yet the Good Samaritan still has a problem of his own. Even when competence is restrained by compassion, the prospect of the multitude of those who can be helped is daunting. Compassion must be circumscribed, just as competence is restrained. The circumscription does not mean any diminution of human feeling, but instead its universalization. Each case must be treated with a fullness compatible with the possibility that another case will receive treatment in the future. This entails a repudiation of the futile and a skepticism about the marginal. It demands an intensity in prevention of disease and in control of its vehemence, as the Hippocratic writings say, so that "rationing" is done by anticipating and avoiding the costly critical incidents. Again, the ambiguity of disease and medicine is managed by affirming that all should be cared for, but each proportionately not only to his or her need but to the needs of those yet to come for help.

The noble ethics of service are revived by this imperative. In the era of the new medicine, it is impossible to implement a proportionate compassion without reforming the institutions of care and the practice of medicine. Samaritans do not travel the roads alone, and hostels are inadequate to house the technologies of modern medicine. Compassion today is delivered, for better or worse, within complex institutional structures and surrounded by intricate forms of practice and financing. Dedication to service can no longer be an individual endeavor, it must be a corporate effort. The profession must critically examine forms of care and practice that restrict access. Entrepreneurial medicine demands the closest scrutiny. Structures of reimbursement and physician payment deserve radical revision. In general, dedication to competent and compassionate service requires duties to political and policy activities.

These duties must lead the profession in a direction it has not enthusiastically taken in the past, namely, away from protection of its self-interest. The slow growth of Lockean rights in medicine has promoted a perception that physicians as such have exclusive dominion over the world of healing. By this perception, the knowledge called medicine is theirs; extensive domains of intervention are theirs alone; even, in a metaphorical way, disease is theirs. Reform of institutions and practice in order to promote compassionate service may require a retreat from some of these claims. This will be difficult, not merely because it may entail some financial peril, but because it may conflict with the other traditional imperative, restrained competence. Allowing other practitioners into the field of care, giving more independence to patients, relaxing the rigidity of scientific investigation in order to make drugs more quickly available, all these raise questions about competence. The retreat from Lockean rights must itself involve the promotion and support of competence in places and persons outside the profession. It requires collaboration with those who are outside the traditional nobility of medicine: nurses, technicians, advocacy groups, patients—even ethicists.

The ethicists, of course, have made their appearance. From

the day Belding Scribner dialyzed Clyde Shields, persons from the disciplines of divinity and philosophy have seen fit to comment on medicine's behavior. Certainly, the long history of medicine has been accompanied by moral comment: doctors were assailed from the pulpit; lists of doctors' sins were compiled; satirists, the moralists of the past, ridiculed the pretensions and impotence of physicians. Catholic theologians and Jewish rabbis included medicine within the strictures of natural and Talmudic law. Medical men themselves, like the Scot John Gregory in the eighteenth century, applied the norms of moral philosophy to the work and character of physicians. A few scholars in moral theology, such as the Catholic Gerald Kelly and the Episcopalian Joseph Fletcher, had written on morality in medicine. Still, until the 1960s, the persons called bioethicists—scholars who devoted all their attention to the moral dimensions of medicine—were unknown. When they did appear, they perceived that the new medicine raised questions that went beyond the purview of physicians' education, experience, and competence, questions frequently summarized under the rubric "who lives? who dies? who decides?" Matters of life and death, and competency to determine their time frame, have always belonged to theology and philosophy.

The early literature of bioethics explored the new issues raised by selection of patients for dialysis and transplantation, the determination of death by neurological criteria, the use of human beings as experimental subjects. Discussions about medical paternalism and patient rights were moved to the philosophical plane. The capabilities of genetics and of reproductive technologies were probed. The occasional article or book about moral issues in medicine became a torrent of literature as theological and philosophical scholars learned medical language and acquainted themselves with clinical activities. Institutes and centers were founded, and almost every medical school in the United States appointed faculty to teach and research medical ethics. Commissions were established by Congress to study many of these issues in depth and to recommend public policy.

Close attention is now given by these scholars to very technical questions. The transplantation of fetal cells, for example, for the cure of diabetes and of neurological diseases has been analyzed in depth by ethicists who know not only ethical theory but neuroscience, at least sufficiently to write respectably about this complex problem. The ethical implications of mapping the human genome, or of germ-cell therapy, are discussed confidently by ethicists. Some issues, such as forgoing life support or cardiopulmonary resuscitation, have undergone such detailed analysis that, for many ethicists, they are the equivalent of the general internist's familiarity with hypertension or upper respiratory infection. They know the problem inside and out and debate it fluently with clinicians in intensive-care units, with ethics committees, and with legal counsel.

What has this new and vigorous discipline (called medical ethics as often as bioethics) to do with the ancient and lasting traditions we have described? Does its close, informed analysis of a variety of issues in medical science and health care belong in the same line? Does it replace them, much as scientific medicine replaced the speculative and empirical medicine of the past? Can its arguments be justified by reference to the traditions, or do the generalities of the tradition merely obscure the clear lines of the ethicists' arguments? Should, or can, the new medical ethics attempt to reform medical institutions or fashion more humane physicians than did the old ethics?

These are questions that ethicists must clarify for themselves and for their audiences, professional and lay. I have my own answer, tentative though it is, and the ambiguity of the Asklepian snake is the key to my formulation. Medicine and its practice is radically ambiguous and, in my opinion, ethics is disciplined reflection on ambiguity. Ethics are generated by the startled encounter of two cherished values facing each other in apparent opposition. One of the earliest recorded documents in ethics is a Greek list of diametrically opposed principles, attributed to the rhetorician Gorgias and called "The Double Arguments." Similarly, one of the earliest recorded debates about ethics portrays Socrates confronting Euthyphro, who believes that the virtue of piety, which should oblige him to revere his father, also obliges him to prosecute his father for homicide. Socrates makes Euthyphro wonder whether a single virtue can give rise to such apparently conflicting duties.

I am certainly not the first to assert that ethics is about ambiguity in life. Many philosophers and theologians have proposed and defended this precept. Thinkers as different as Simone de Beauvoir and Reinhold Niebuhr have held some version of the thesis and have come to quite different conclusions about the meaning of life. But outside of learned dissertations the hypothesis sounds rather banal. Many a person, reasonable and respectable, has concluded that ethical issues are often intrinsically ambiguous and so insoluble. They maintain a skeptical stance toward all ethical discourse; after all, there are two sides to every question.

Ambiguity, so much a part of human life, is cheapened if we think of it as merely describing the confusion, doubt, and uncertainty that accompany many human problems. It also describes something more profound. It has an objective meaning which, the Oxford English Dictionary notes, is historically prior to the subjective one. It means "capable of being understood in more than one way." This defines more than confusion; it defines reality. The etymology of the word, from the Latin *ambigere* (to walk around, in several directions), suggests an even deeper meaning. Human affairs may have several outcomes, may carry diverse intentions, and may wander away from human control.

An English philosopher, G. J. Warnock, finds in this deep ambiguity the meaning of ethics. He suggests that what we call ethics is the attempt to contribute to the betterment of "the human predicament," and that predicament is "inherently such that things are liable to go badly." They are so liable because human rationality and human sympathy are, by their nature, limited in depth and scope. It is the proper business of ethics, Warnock claims, "to make us more rational in the judicious pursuit of our interests and ends; to expand our sympathies, or better, to reduce the liability to damage inherent in their natural tendency to be narrowly restricted."[6] We have seen that medicine is radically ambiguous in this sense: it can go badly wrong even as it aims to heal. It can bring great benefits at great price, and improve some at cost to others. The mysterious snake, fascinating and repellent, became its symbol. So, likewise, ethics are about ambiguity. Ethics do not merely announce ambiguity; they warn in order to prevent or at least reduce the chance of "things going badly." They work at expanding rationality and sympathy, stretching them to cover the new case, the strange situation, the threatening possibility.

Without becoming too academic, I think one can affirm that ethics are about ambiguity and at the same time affirm that ethical argument can come to closure on certain questions. It is through this approach that the great traditions of medical ethics and the work of the modern medical ethicist come together. The traditions remind us forcibly of the ambiguities of life as they show themselves in the crises of illness and the work of healing. Although expressed in the idiom of the times, these ambiguities have been remarkably similar throughout quite different eras of Western culture.

Disguising or forgetting ambiguity is one of the perils of the moral life. It is much more comfortable to see life as a seamless whole, or as ordered by a single rule, than as inherently ambiguous. The "one-issue politics" we often deplore arises from "one-principle ethics." Religious zealots and political fanatics follow but one rule, whatever it may be. Whatever does not conform to that rule, or follow that principle, must be ignored or destroyed. The work of healing is also in constant danger of becoming univocal, of speaking with only one voice about its accomplishments. In yielding to that temptation, it falsifies itself and deceives others.

Resolutions of new problems are attained by elevating to consciousness the precise features generated by modern technology and social conditions, by understanding how these challenge the traditions by favoring one or another side of the intrinsic ambiguities. The resolutions will be more or less reasonable to the extent that they preserve the positive values of the traditions without failing to recognize the negative. For example, the expansion of scientific and clinical competence into the new areas of genetic diagnosis and therapy highlights the ambiguity surrounding the identity of the patient. Resolutions offered by bioethicists to the particular problems in this area must (as they generally have) favor the relief of particular presenting patients over the eradication of future disease in patients not yet existing. That is, therapeutics should have priority over eugenics. Prevention of disease remains a desired goal, but not at the price of allowing competence to stray from its duties toward patients into dangerous regions of social engineering. In so doing, competence can lose its identity.

Contemporary bioethicists, then, are not creating new ethics for medicine. They are bringing the old ethics into a new era and asking them questions about problems that they could not have imagined in detail but did anticipate in outline. The new problems about genetics, transplantation, neuroscience, provision of services, and the like are new in their technical, social, and economic detail. They are old in the ethical outlines that were prefigured within the traditions: the outlines of limits to competence, finitude of compassion, protection of privilege, and propriety over skills. The new language of bioethics, summed up in the mantra "beneficence, nonmaleficence, autonomy, and justice," becomes under close examination little more than the modern version of the old traditions. These words shed little theoretical illumination on the new problems and do even less to resolve them. But if one goes behind the vocabulary to the traditions and their ambiguity, one can glimpse their true meaning: they call to mind the tension inherent in illness and healing and the provisional nature of any resolution to any current problem.

We have noted that one of the perils of the moral life consists in ignoring or forgetting its ambiguities. In recent decades it has become common to refer to the progress of modern medicine as a succession of miracles. Penicillin was heralded as a miracle, as was the introduction of open-heart surgery. The eradication of polio by immunization and the transplantation and implantation of human hearts were described as miracles. A public television series entitled "Managing Our Miracles" described one after another the technological and scientific breakthroughs, then showed how each had raised significant ethical, social, and economic problems.

The description of medical progress as miraculous is a form of rhetorical entrapment. It spreads a luminous but obscuring fog over the ambiguities of that progress and of medicine itself. The term "miracle," although it has lost in our secular era its original denotation of a divine intervention in nature, retains the connotations of "wondrous, marvelous, admirable." It is hard to think of a bad miracle or one with ambiguous effects. "Managing Our Miracles" had it right, however: it noted that the "miracles" were not unambiguously beneficial. It is perhaps one of the handicaps of bioethics that it must do its work in the environment of medical miracles, for critics of miracles are usually unwelcome.

We have taken a long voyage through the moral mythology and history of medicine. The next stage in that voyage is a brief stop at a myth that may have been history (although I am skeptical about that). It tells of a miracle of medicine that was a miracle in the original sense of the word. Twin brothers from Asia Minor, Cosmos and Damien, practiced medicine without fee. In A.D. 303 they were martyred for their Christian faith and came to be venerated throughout Christendom as the patron saints of physicians. Legend credits them with the first transplantation surgery. The saintly physicians appeared in a vision to a man sleeping in the church built in their honor in Rome. The man suffered from a gangrenous leg and had come to the church to petition the saints to intercede. From heaven the brothers heard the man's prayer, and while he slept amputated the leg and replaced it with a "healthy" leg taken from a corpse. The patient was white, the donor was black (as was the case in one of the first heart transplants in South Africa!). Presumably the sleeping recipient did not give "informed consent" nor did the cadaver have a signed donor card. The holy physicians saved the life of their patient and left him with a miscegenetic limb. The saints performed a miracle, for there was no natural way in which a limb from the corpse (unless he was brain dead but still on a respirator, which the story does not indicate) would thrive on their patient. But their miracle was marred and inept in several ways; while its efficacy derived from a divine source, its performance was by human skills.

Presumably even saints can be clumsy. The work of the holy physicians suggests a good way to view the miracles of modern medicine: as wondrous in comparison with the alternatives, but ambiguously so.

Now the snakes of Asklepios and the saints of Jesus Christ come together: both were believed to have power and to perform miracles. At the same time, human skill is involved. Asklepios learned how to use herbs as medicine; Cosmos and Damien are depicted with primitive surgical instruments. They knew how to resect and connect (and, amazingly, to anastomose blood vessels, a skill credited to sixteenth-century Dr. Ambroise Paré!). Both the pagan and the Christian myths suggest a mysterious mix of human art and supernatural power.

One author, describing the votive tablets placed in the Asklepieona by individuals cured of their diseases, links the ancient and Christian miracles of cure:

> The cures recorded in the tablets also represent an enigma, though of a more general kind. They raise the same problem as most of the "miraculous cures" at the many Christian places of pilgrimage in southern and central Europe. They are "miraculous" only insofar as every cure, every happy ending to a situation implying the possibility of an unhappy one, is a miracle. Wherever a living creature—who might equally be called a dying creature—is gravely ill, every turn for the better involves an element of mystery, even when the physician has recognized and eliminated the cause of sickness. For the physician cannot act alone: side by side with his outside

intervention something inside the patient must lend a helping hand if a cure is to be accomplished . . . Thus, the cures [at the Asklepeona] are no more mysterious than the cures effected anywhere else: healing itself is the mystery.[7]

Present-day physicians with all the technology of modern medicine participate in that mystery. No matter how much we know about antibodies, osmolality, immunoglobulins, or any of the other revealed mysteries of the body, at the heart of the science of medicine the mystery remains. The patient also participates in the mystery, for even without the science the patient knows himself or herself intimately. Today others participate in the mystery, for they contribute to bringing patients and physicians together in the settings for care. Thus, the modern miracles are coproduced by a different cast than the ancient miracles: in those, the god and the saint, or the snake, worked together; in contemporary miracles, the patient, the physicians, and the multitude of providers cooperate.

We frequently hear that physicians "play God" when they make decisions about life and death. The phrase is supposed to suggest arrogance. Yet it is a dim echo of ancient beliefs that in all healing, God is active. The rabbis of ancient Judaism justified the use of physicians by proposing that they healed by the power of God. Ambroise Paré, the father of modern surgery (the one who discovered how to anastomose unmiraculously), adopted the motto "I treat, God heals." In a more secular era, the flippant phrase "playing God" is about all that remains of that ancient belief. Yet with it we remind ourselves of the mystery of medicine. Two admonitions of the Greek medical tradition put the godlike role of the physician in proper context. In the Hippocratic writings we find the words "Transport wisdom into medicine and medicine into wisdom, for the physician who loves wisdom is like a god."[8] The wisdom of the Greeks was an appreciation of the potential and the limits of life; hubris was a violation not only of divine law but of human limits. The wisdom that is to be transported into medicine is the sense of limitation that restrains competence from overreaching. It is this appreciation that creates the similarity between human and divine judgment.

In an inscription on the pediment of the Asklepieon of Athens, the following words appear:

> Physicians must be like gods:
> bringing benefit to all alike,
> the rich and poor, men and women,
> friend and enemy.[9]

These words are a pagan intimation of the lesson of the Good Samaritan. In pagan fashion they compare the works and character of the physician who cares for all in need to the work of the gods which benefits all mankind. In the parable of the Good Samaritan, Jesus orders his followers to consider as neighbors not just those who are friends and coreligionists, but those who are joined as needy and helper. In this way the helpers become "children of your Father which is in heaven; for he maketh his sun to rise on the evil and on the good and sendeth rain on the just and on the unjust" (Matt. 5:45). The nobility of medicine bowed to "our lords, the sick" and acknowledged a duty to serve. The possessive individualism that grew up around modern medicine was persuaded to cede its rights of absolute propriety before a democracy of cooperative rights.

In all of these traditions ambiguity is present. It is perhaps best expressed by the nuances of the phrases "playing God," or "being like God." The physician is not God but in a certain respect must imitate God. That respect is the intention of impartial beneficence. But the imitation is imperfect; it is an actor's playing of a beneficent God and as such it is limited, finite, imperfect, and fallible. In the more modern imagery of rights and democracy, it involves the negotiating and compromises that are necessary to a democracy made up of individuals each enjoying inviolable rights. The ethics of medicine, in their great traditions and in their contemporary work of what we have called interstitial resolutions, are an effort to make the best of an ambiguous reality, always poised between death and life, compassion and exploitation, possessiveness and generosity, dominance and autonomy. Ethics are the human effort to catch hold of those human events and occasions that "are liable to go badly" and turn them to our good as best we can.

Chapter 7

Humanities Are the Hormones

The odd phrase "Humanities are the hormones" comes from the last lecture delivered by the man who, above all others, united in his mind and work the humanities and medical science—Sir William Osler. We have already met Sir William as the embodiment of the noble ethos of medicine. In 1919, several months before his death, Oxford's Regius Professor of Medicine was elected president of the British Classical Society. He called his presidential lecture, "The Old Humanities and the New Science," a title that obviously inspired the title of this book. In the course of this speech about the ways in which scientific education and the humanities should inform each other, Sir William told his audience of classical scholars:

> You secrete materials which do for society at large what the thyroid gland does for the individual. The humanities are the hormones . . . The humanities bring the student into contact with the minds who gave us the philosophies, the models of our literature, the ideals of democratic freedom, the fine and technical arts, the fundamentals of science, the basis of our law . . . into contact with the dead who never die, with those immortal lives "not of now, nor of yesterday, but who always are." [1]

Why call humanities the hormones? Sir William exploits the etymology of the word "hormone," which in ancient Greek means "to set in motion, urge, push on." He suggests by this metaphor that the work of classical scholars energizes the intellectual life of society, just as the thyroid gland energizes the intellectual life of an individual. He says:

> Man's body is a humming hive of working cells each with its specific function, all under the control of the brain and heart, and all dependent on materials called hormones . . . which lubricate the wheels of life. For example, remove the thyroid gland just below the Adam's apple, and you deprive man of the lubricants which enable his thought engines to work, and gradually the stored acquisitions of his mind cease to be available and within a year he sinks into dementia . . . The paragon of animals is transformed into a shapeless caricature of humanity.[2]

When Sir William was speaking, endocrinology was in its infancy. Adrenaline was the first hormone to be isolated in 1902 and the generic name "hormone" was chosen several years later with the help of the professor of Greek at Gonville and Caius College, Cambridge. E. H. Starling, lecturing in 1905 before the Royal College of Physicians, noted that "chemical messengers—or hormones as we might call them—have to be carried to the organ which they affect by means of the blood stream, and the recurring physiological needs of the organism must determine their repeated production and circulation throughout the body."[3]

By the time the Regius Professor was lecturing in 1919, many hormones had been identified—including thyroxine, which E. C. Kendall had discovered in 1914. Thus, Sir William was describing for his classical scholars (W. T. Vesey, the classicist who had named the "hormones," might have been in the audience) the course of hypothyroidism or myxedema, a clinical condition long known to be caused by deficiency of iodine, but now understood more fundamentally as a hormonal dysfunction. In primary hypothyroidism, decreased or absent secretion of thyroxine leads to an accumulation of mucopolysaccharide in connective tissue. The result is weakness, lethargy, dry skin, edema, cramps, constipation; more to Sir William's purposes, there is also a mental effect. In the words of a modern medical text: "Hearing impairment, somnolence, decreased memory and ability to calculate may occur. These may lead to psychological withdrawal and paranoia. The term myxedema madness has been used to describe this syndrome, which can be mistaken for dementia."[4] Sir William, acute clinician though he was, did not know the precise etiology of myxedema madness. But its clinical manifestation, together with its newly discovered linkage to the hormone thyroxine, gave him matter for a fine metaphor, "Humanities are the hormones."

His thesis is that humanistic studies—the classics, history, philosophy—energize or, as he says, lubricate, the intelligence of society. Without their stimulation human society dries up, becomes mentally vacant and wandering. Humanities are to society, Sir William claims, as hormones are to the body. However, in *The Old Humanities and the New Science,* Sir William was not arguing for the humanities; there was no need for that at Oxford in 1919. He was complaining that higher education ignored science. He exclaimed, "The School of Humane Letters excites wonder in the extent and variety of the knowledge demanded . . . but this wonder pales before gaping astonishment at what is not there . . . The sources of the new science that has made a new world are practically ignored."[5]

Seventy years after his lecture, the humanities no longer hold primacy in secondary and higher education. Occasional advocates, like William Bennett, Allan Bloom, and E. D. Hirsch, decry the decay of the humanities; academic programs in the humanities, such as Saint John's Great Books curriculum, are so rare as to elicit admiring notice by educators. Science majors march unimpeded through experiments, formulas, and equations, with at best a bothersome bivouac in an occasional Great Literature or Western Civilizations course. The university departments that profess the humanities have often become enclaves of "critical studies" that are so arcane as to repel the broad-minded inquirer, to say nothing of the scientist.

Education for medicine at all levels (undergraduate preparation, medical school, and residency training) is, as it should be, scientific and clinical. It is almost totally insulated from the humanities. As Charles Odegaard has stated—or, rather, understated—"The humanities and social sciences are not the disciplines in the university setting with which physicians tend to be more familiar."[6] And Eric Cassell remarks:

Always a concern, early in the post-Flexnerian era the debate over the proper educational background for physicians resumed, and the tension between humanism and scientism has continued ever since . . . Commissions and reports, from the late 1920's to the present, have championed liberal education over narrow vocationalism. Nonetheless, continuing surveys of medical school requirements testify to the lack of impact of such recommendations.[7]

One of many such reports, *The General Professional Education of Physicians in the Twenty-First Century,* issued by the Association of American Medical Colleges in 1984, encourages students preparing for admission to medical school to avoid premature specialization in the sciences and to avail themselves of advanced courses in the humanities. The ghost of Sir William lurks behind these words, "By the time their college studies are completed these students often have forfeited the intellectual challenges and rewards that study in the humanities could have afforded."[8]

I return to Sir William's metaphor in order to reflect on the relationship between biomedical science and the humanities in the context of modern medical education, practice, and policy. Up to this point in our voyage through the myth and history of medicine, we have traveled the paths of ethos and ethics in the world of medicine. But these paths cross a large landscape of ideas and events. The map of the large landscape is drawn by history and philosophy, two humanistic disciplines that are of vital importance for medicine. Our use of historical incidents and personages, as well as our reference to certain ethical notions, must be fitted into the larger framework of those disciplines.

There are faculty in medical history and in the philosophy of medicine. Their work needs no apology. Sound scholarship and competent teaching issue from the relatively few humanities programs in schools of medicine; their contribution is from time to time acknowledged and appreciated by medical educators and students. Still, the place of the medical humanities does need to be explained. We "humanists" must publicly announce what we do, why we do it, and, above all, why what we do is good for medicine. Being humanists, dedicated to the word in speech and on the page, we are not shy about doing so. Many humanists, physicians, and other scholars have reasoned eloquently. Sir William, Edmund Pellegrino, Charles Odegaard, Eric Cassell, and others have argued that the humanities contribute to the making of educated, humane, and compassionate physicians. Now I add my voice to the chorus.

The endocrine metaphor is still, I think, an apt one around which to develop this argument. Sir William referred to thyroid hormone, not only because it was one of the few whose action was understood in his day, but also because deficiency in its action actually seemed to shrivel intelligence. It was, then, a wonderful metaphor with which to make his point to classical scholars: without their endeavors, he asserted, social intelligence would wither. We might agree with him and say that medicine, without the humanities, is as desiccated as the mummy of Mr. Bentham. Or we might extend his metaphor. The secretions of another endocrine gland, the adrenal cortex, provide another perspective. I might paraphrase Sir William, "Humanities are the corticoids." Not as euphonious or alliterative, but pertinent for two reasons that are suggested in a physiology text:

> The production of glucocorticoids and mineralo-corticoids by the adrenal cortex is stimulated by ACTH from the pituitary, which in turn is stimulated by impulses from the hypo-

thalamus . . . The adrenal cortex is essential to life because it is largely by its means that the body succeeds in adapting itself to constant changes in the environment. [10]

The hormones of the adrenal cortex, then, provide a fine example of the complex interrelation between hormones and nervous system and the exquisite routing of chemical messages between distant sites. They also contribute in a significant way to homeostasis, the essential balance within the body and between the body and its environs. We could also note the adrenal contribution to sexuality in its physical, physiological, and psychological aspects (and if we included the medullary hormones, the impact on the human psyche and emotions). Even restricting ourselves to the cortical hormones, we are struck by their essential and complex role, more often than not demonstrated by their deficiencies. A medical text notes that "clinical disorders of the adrenal glands are relatively uncommon, but when present, result in some of the most striking syndromes in clinical medicine." [11]

My thesis is that the humanities—in particular history of medicine, philosophy of medicine, and medical ethics—are, in a way, the chemical messengers that course through the complicated institution of medicine and enable it to respond to the constantly changing scientific, technological, social, and economic environment. Like hormonal secretions, they are present only in minute quantities in the vast organism of medicine, and in another resemblance, their release into that organism is pulsatile, stimulated by challenge. The humanities are the agents of homeostasis in medicine.

This is a bold thesis. Indeed, given the modest place

occupied by the medical humanities today, it would seem to imply that modern medicine is afflicted with a social version of Addison's disease or Cushing's disease, both the results of serious hormone deficiency. Let that implication pass (though there may be something in it) and permit me to argue my position.

History and philosophy are disciplines with long lineages; their appearance varies with ages, authors, scholarly traditions and fads. It is perilous to generalize. Yet I will risk saying that, despite the multiplicity of theories and definitions of these disciplines, history is inevitably preoccupied with memory and philosophy is incessantly engrossed with meaning. Each can be pursued as an independent discipline, with its own canon of research; each can be studied in isolation from the other and in isolation from current, actual events. Each can produce sound and brilliant scholarship, uncompelled by the demands of immediate relevance.

When these humanities live within the world of medicine and the biomedical sciences, however, they become, as it were, relatives in a family of ideas, institutions, and practices. They participate in the continual conversation of that family. The conversation is most often scientific, technical, and clinical, but on occasion it is interrupted by a question about origins, evolution, meaning, and value. At such moments the historian and the philosopher of medicine can put in a word. Sometimes their contribution is only a curiosity—it is fascinating to know, for example, how hormones were found and by whom, or to listen for a short while to how disease and illness should be conceptually distinguished.

At other times the contribution of the historian and the

philosopher is much more. It is sometimes essential to understanding what is happening or what has gone wrong or what ought to be done. The historical narrative or the philosophical reflection redirects the conversation or elevates it to a different plane. In this sense the humanities are like the hormones, chemical messengers that affect end organs far from their source; the humanities send messages to the practices, policies, and institutions of medicine and science, messages about memory and meaning that may not be noticed for themselves but that stimulate and regulate activities. These messages from a remote source, like the steroid hormones, effect the balance between the inner activities of medicine and science and the outer environment of society and culture.

Again, these are bold, even rash, assertions. No one would question such claims if the subject were the relationship between biochemistry and medicine or between molecular biology and medicine: it is clear that these sciences are dominant contributors to the conversations that make up biomedicine. People can think and talk and perform excellent science and competent clinical medicine without hearing a word of history or philosophy. Similarly, the great medical institutions that provide health care or education or do research seem to carry on their business without much help from the humanists. (Indeed, several years ago Rockefeller University dismissed its entire philosophy faculty, some of whom were world renowned, as superfluous to a biomedical research university.) How, then, can I be so vain as to claim that the humanities function hormone-like in the organism of medicine?

Historical memory and philosophical meaning are incessantly at work within and throughout the enterprise of medicine. Just as cortisol constantly functions within the organism to affect carbohydrate, protein, lipid, and water metabolism, so the current practices and institutions of medicine function because of the way in which the past secretes into the present, and meanings and values secrete into behavior and policy. Endocrine secretions function constantly, but are stimulated only when the feedback mechanism signals imbalance; similarly, memory and meaning move from a tacit to an overt presence within medicine when external forces and internal imbalances appear. Then medicine must call up its memories and reflect on its values. This is the time for the humanities. Odegaard puts the point eloquently:

> Leafing through the pages of the past, seeing the different goals for human living that have been put forth in other times and places . . . the humanist is often led to raise the normative questions: what are the best choices? what are the preferred ends? . . . He often brings to light even the hidden values which this and earlier generations have accepted for their lives and enables men the better to discern the value consequences of changes in society.[12]

Medicine, as science, as practice, and as social institution, has undergone a vast transition over the past forty years. Much has been written about the changes, and senior physicians can describe them in vivid terms. All of those changes challenge the fundamental values that medical memory and medical meaning reveal. Among the manifold values the most important are the duty to benefit the patient, the responsibility for competence, the obligation to care for the sick, the utility of research, and the integrity of scientific discovery. Throughout its history, medicine at its best has been praised for scrupulously competent clinical care; fidelity, even friendship, toward patients; honest, rigorous science; educated concern for the health of the public; and a generous willingness to welcome the needy sick. Medicine at its worst has been condemned for obscurantism, faddishness, venality—for being monopolistic of its benefits and dangerous in its power. We have already reflected on these persistent themes.

In all the changes that have marked medicine in the last four decades, these best and worst qualities struggle for control. As science achieves heights of intellectual mastery, dishonesty creeps in. As therapy achieves heights of clinical efficacy, impersonalism and venality appear. One need not be profoundly read in the humanities to condemn the occasions on which medicine's worse side wins these conflicts: their iniquity is manifest. The problem posed to the humanities in an era of change is how to recognize medicine's perennial values in the welter of innovation, and how to acknowledge the new values that innovation requires in order to be not merely new medicine, but good medicine. When one reflects on these questions, medicine's memory about its best and worst and medicine's reflection on the meaning of best and worst become indispensable. This is how the new medicine and the old ethics must converse with each other.

There are many notable examples of this remembering and reflection. I recall two in which I was personally involved. The first was the debate over the ethics of using human subjects in biomedical research. In the late 1960s, biomedical research was flourishing. Then several research projects were accused of unethical use of human subjects. The study of the natural history of hepatitis at Willowbrook (New York) State Hospital, which involved retarded children, and the study of the natural history of syphilis in a poor, rural, black population in Tuskegee, Alabama, were the most notorious. Even apart from these widely publicized cases, there was a general impression that scientific research was being carried out with a certain insouciance about the rights and welfare of its human subjects.

In the next few years the thinking about involvement of human subjects gradually changed. The new formulation was created by recalling many events—some praiseworthy, such as Walter Reed's yellow fever investigations, some evil, such as the Nazi concentration camp experiments. Reflection on those events, on current practices, and on the exigencies of modern science produced an ethic of research with human subjects in which certain values, such as autonomy and beneficence, stood side by side with the classical utilitarian justification. Historians and philosophers were stimulated to action (except that it sounds vaguely obscene, we might stay with our hormonal metaphor by saying "to secretion") by a serious imbalance in a major segment of biomedical science. Their contributions, together with those of many scientists and policy makers, restored balance. Research involving human subjects continues today with prominent safeguards for the rights and welfare of its participants and without notable detriment to scientific progress.

A second challenge to the organism of medicine came from

its achievement of life-sustaining technologies. Scribner's development of chronic hemodialysis was among the first of these technologies, together with the evolution of artificially assisted respiration from the negative-pressure Drinker tank in the 1950s to the positive-pressure ventilators of today. These technologies did wonders in staving off imminent death. At the same time, they made it possible, as the common phrase puts it, to prolong dying. Karen Ann Quinlan became a symbol of this ambivalence: Was her continued life in a persistent vegetative state a benefit to her? Was the refusal of her physician to cease life-supporting treatment an act of fidelity?

For a decade philosophers, theologians, and historians probed these questions of memory and meaning. At one point the writings of a sixteenth-century casuist, Domenico Bañez, helped the President's Commission for the Study of Ethical Problems in Medicine to understand the vexed meaning of "ordinary and extraordinary" care. A phalanx of contemporary philosophers subsequently provided distinctions and clarifications that Bañez had not thought of.[13] Today, while certain difficult questions remain unsettled, many of the ancient values of medicine, such as fidelity to the patient and the duty to prolong life, have been clarified. Certain new values, such as the autonomy of the patient, have come into focus. The medical humanities have helped to produce the concepts and the logic that allow medicine to understand how these technologies can contribute to its best purposes.

A dramatic challenge to medicine's memory and meaning now faces us in the AIDS epidemic. American medicine had enjoyed a long respite from epidemic disease. During that respite medicine evolved into a more technological, more scientific, more organizationally and financially elaborate enterprise than it had been when epidemic disease was a constant menace. That evolution has made it possible to isolate and identify the viral agent of this new epidemic and to specify the routes whereby it travels. At the same time, that evolution has dimmed the awareness of certain features of epidemic disease that our medical forebears knew only too well: that control is a political and social problem, not a medical one; that duty to serve the sick has to be balanced against risk; that access to care can be marred by discrimination for class, race, or finances; that sickness brings not only suffering but stigma. Medical theory maintained for many centuries that epidemic disease arose from the conjunction of many influences—celestial, meteorological, geographic—at a certain time and place. That theory was called the "epidemic constitution." Even though it was incorrect, it was a reminder that the complex interaction of many elements creates epidemics. In an age in which microorganisms were discovered to be the agents of infectious disease, we have forgotten the outmoded theory of the epidemic constitution. AIDS is forcing us to rediscover it in a new form with the recognition that the virus moves from person to person because of complex behaviors, beliefs, and social structures.

These are truths that must be extracted from the deep memory of medicine. As they are recalled, they must be rethought in light of ancient and new values in medicine, the ancient duty to serve and the new duty to be just in allocation of service. The concept of rights of patients, never as familiar in Lockean medicine as were the rights of doctors, becomes a central one in understanding the AIDS epidemic, in formulating policies about it and in caring for its victims. Again, history and philosophy are stimulated by an imbalance: scientific, technological medicine does not respond satisfactorily to a disease spread primarily by engaging in stigmatized behavior. Epidemic lethal disease is not well managed by a health-care system designed by free enterprise and dominated by entrepreneurial institutions. Standards of responsibility are eroded by the perception of serious danger in carrying out one's duty. In all of these ways the institution and practices of medicine come under stress, stimulating a pulsatile release of memories and meanings that can bring it back to that balance in which all who are in need of care receive it from competent and confident practitioners, a balance in which the threats of disease are met by proportionate defenses.

Earlier in this book we have seen major shifts entering the institution of medicine. Where the physician was once the dominant actor, the patient-physician relationship the dominant scenario, and diagnosis and therapy the dominant script, we now confront a cast in which physicians, a multitude of other providers, and newly empowered patients share billing. The patient-physician relationship remains the main act, but it is preceded and followed by equally important acts: scientific and clinical research beforehand, and the social and financial implications of care afterward. The new diagnostics and therapeutics raise the question "Who is the patient?" as the populations envisioned by genetics and transplantation come into view. To the roles of diagnosis and therapy, the new script adds prominent parts for prevention and, alas, for rationing. The traditional ethic of physician benevolence and fidelity, which fitted the old play, must be expanded by principles of autonomy and justice. Historical memory and philosophical reflection are essential contributors to the ongoing revision of the drama of medicine. The Hippocratic, Cabotean, and Samaritanian ethics come onstage again, but in modern dress, speaking in contemporary language.

Historical memory brings to these new scripts honesty about the past. The history of medicine is a record of scientific discovery, clinical triumph, and personal sacrifice; it is also, as we have seen, a history of obscurantism, dogmatism, and greed. Asklepios, remarkable healer though he was, yielded to "the lure of gold." This darker side warns us to expect similar responses in contemporary crises. Likewise, the revered value of service to the patient, motivating as it does much sacrifice and effecting much good, can mask self-interest and selfishness in the profession. The Samaritan may ignore the victims when they become too numerous and too unprofitable. The noble ethos of compassion may build its defensive fortress. These myths and histories must be remembered. The philosophical analysis of altruism and self-interest, responsibility to self and to others, duty to patient and to society, must inform the entire range of response to scientific progress, technological achievement, insidious disease.

Still other challenges await medicine: commercialism, the power inherent in genetic and reproductive manipulation, the possibilities of and obstacles to prevention of disease. Each calls for clarification, reaffirmation, revision, and sometimes abandonment of medicine's memories and meaning. Each requires clarification of concepts such as benefit, utility, responsibility, autonomy, for this new set of scientific, technical, social, and economic circumstances. Value concepts are as important as scientific concepts for the life of medicine.

A contemporary essayist, writing about the importance of historical memory in modern societies, posits that societies "need to connect with their past in order to deal with their present: to make moral sense of the past in order to possess moral confidence in the future."[14] The phrase that urges making "moral sense of the past in order to possess moral confidence in the future" eloquently expresses the hormonal function of the humanities in medicine. Medicine is a highly complex reality, made up of trained persons, in a variety of roles, performing a multitude of functions—and of untrained persons seeking their attention. If this complicated reality is thought of as an organism, the equilibrium of its many components can frequently be threatened. Response to such threats must be rapid and efficient, but at the same time preserve the essential structures whereby the reality can be recognized. Those structures derive from the history of medicine, as the structures of the organism derive from its genetics. The ability to distinguish the essential structures from the accidental and adventitious ones derives from philosophical reflection, much as the sensitive neural regulation and feedback control of the hypothalamic-pituitary system discerns the level and target of neuroendocrine response.

History and philosophy of medicine give moral meaning to the past; moral confidence in the future can only be achieved by the scientists, administrators, and practitioners of medicine who understand its moral meaning. It is their responsibility to revise the institutions and practices created in the past without loss of moral meaning. A highly scientific medicine that reaches only a privileged minority is morally deficient. An extraordinarily competent corps of practitioners that deals only with cure and knows nothing of prevention is morally deficient. A cost-effective system of care that shuts out the dying or the elderly or the poor is morally deficient. Those responsible for the revision of medicine's past to meet its future must have confidence that they can make those revisions without sacrifice of its essential values and with the readiness to incorporate new values.

Of course, many fluids course through the body of medicine: science and clinical skill, education and health-care administration, specialties, self-regulation, publishing, politics. The corticoids of the humanities are but a part of the whole. Surely medicine's response to challenges derives from all parts of its complex body. Among these the products of the humanities, memory and meaning, are particularly vital to its continued life. History and philosophy of medicine are not extrinsic to medicine; rather, in the words of our physiology text, they are "essential to life because [by them] the body adapts itself to constant changes in the environment."

It is in this sense that we reaffirm Sir William Osler's metaphor: humanities are the hormones. He spoke of the Old Humanities and the New Science. We speak of the New Medicine and the Old Ethics. Whatever the formulation, the powerful technologies and sciences that make up the New Medicine must be given life by a constant flow of memory and meaning.

Notes

Index

Notes

Introduction

1. Leon Wieseltier, "Unlocking the Rabbi's Secrets," *New York Times Book Review*, December 17, 1989, p. 3.

1. Asklepios as Intensivist

1. Renee Fox and Judith Swazy, *The Courage To Fail: A Social View of Organ Transplants and Dialysis* (Chicago: University of Chicago Press, 1974).

2. Shana Alexander, "They Decide Who Lives, Who Dies: Medical Miracle Puts a Burden on a Small Committee," *Life,* November 9, 1962, p. 102.

3. Pindar, *Third Pythian Ode* 3.1–7, 47–60; F. J. Nisetich, ed., *Pindar's Victory Songs* (Baltimore: Johns Hopkins University Press, 1980), pp. 169, 171; translation slightly modified. See also Plato, *Republic* 3.408.

4. Hippocrates, *On the Sacred Disease* 5, ed. and trans. W. H. S. Jones (Cambridge, Mass.: Harvard University Press, 1962); translation occasionally altered.

5. Hippocrates, *Law* 4.

6. Hippocrates, *Precepts* 2.

7. Hippocrates, *Oath*.

8. Sir George Clark, *A History of the Royal College of Physicians of London* (Oxford: Clarendon Press, 1964), I, 99.

9. Roderigo a Castro, *Medicus Politicus* (Hamburg, 1614), pp. 2–4.

10. Ahasverius Fritsch, *Medicus Peccans* (Nuremberg, 1684), p. 2.

11. Chester Burns, "Richard Clarke Cabot and Reformation in American Medical Ethics," *Bulletin of the History of Medicine* 51 (1977): 353–368; quotation on p. 368.

12. Francis Peabody, "The Care of the Patient," *Journal of the American Medical Association* 88 (1927): 877–881; quotation on p. 881.

13. President's Commission for the Study of Ethical Problems in Medicine and in Biomedical and Behavioral Research, *Deciding to Forego Life-Sustaining Treatment* (Washington, D.C.: Government Printing Office, 1983).

14. *New York Times,* September 1, 1988, p. 1.

15. W. T. Friedewald, "Epidemiology of Cardiovascular Disease," J. B. Wyngaarden and L. H. Smith, eds., *Cecil Textbook of Medicine,* 18th ed. (Philadelphia: W. B. Saunders, 1988), p. 180.

16. Michael Bishop, "Oncogenes," in Wyngaarden and Smith, *Cecil Textbook,* pp. 1089, 1092.

17. Rudolf Virchow, *Gesammelte Abhandlungen aus dem Gebiete der Öffentlichen Medicin* (Berlin: Herschwald, 1879), I, 34.

18. Aristotle, *Nicomachean Ethics* 5.9.1137all–16, trans. H. Rackham (Cambridge, Mass.: Harvard University Press, 1962); translation somewhat modified.

2. The Good Samaritan as Gatekeeper

1. Walsh McDermott and David Rogers, "Technology's Consort," *American Journal of Medicine* 74 (1983): 353–358; quotation on p. 353.

2. John Chrysostom, Homily 10 on Heb. 6, 7–8, in Philip Schaff, ed., *The Nicene and Post-Nicene Fathers of the Christian Church,* ser. 1 (New York: Charles Scribner's Sons, 1905–1908), XIV, 417.

3. Henry Sigerist, *Medicine and Human Welfare* (New Haven: Yale University Press, 1941), p. 11.

4. Hippocrates, *On Wounds.* See also Guido Majno, *The Healing Hand: Man and Wound in the Ancient World* (Cambridge, Mass.: Harvard University Press, 1975), pp. 176–200; J. A. Fitzmyer, *The Gospel of Luke,* Anchor Bible (Garden City, N.Y.: Doubleday, 1981), pp. 51–53, 882–890.

5. Immanuel Jakobovits, *Jewish Medical Ethics* (New York: Bloch, 1958), chap. 20.

6. See Norman Daniels, *Just Health Care* (Cambridge: Cambridge University Press, 1985); Daniel Callahan, *Setting Limits* (New York: Simon and Schuster, 1987); Larry Churchill, *Rationing Health Care in America* (Notre Dame: University of Notre Dame Press, 1987).

7. Howard Hiatt, "Protecting the Medical Commons: Who Is Responsible?" *New England Journal of Medicine* 235 (1975): 235–240.

8. See J. M. Eisenberg, "The Internist as Gatekeeper," *Annals of Internal Medicine* 102 (1985): 537–543; M. D. Reagan, "Physicians as Gatekeepers: A Complex Challenge," *New England Journal of Medicine* 317 (1987): 1731–33.

9. Gerald Winslow, *Triage and Justice* (Berkeley: University of California Press, 1982).

10. Paul Ramsey, *Patient as Person* (New Haven: Yale University Press, 1970), pp. 116–118.

11. See A. R. Jonsen, "Organ Transplantation," in Robert Veatch, *Medical Ethics* (Boston: Jones and Bartlett, 1989), pp. 229–253.

12. Alasdair MacIntyre, *Whose Justice, Whose Rationality?* (Notre Dame: University of Notre Dame Press, 1988), p. 395.

13. Ramsey, *Patient as Person*, p. 240.

14. Francis D. Moore, "The Desperate Case: CARE (Costs, Applicability, Research, Ethics)," *Journal of the American Medical Association* 261 (1989): 1483–84.

15. Plato, *Republic* 3.406.

16. Hippocrates, *Art* 8.

17. President's Commission for the Study of Ethical Problems in Medicine and in Biomedical and Behavioral Research, *Deciding to Forego Life-Sustaining Treatment* (Washington, D.C.: Government Printing Office, 1983), pp. 88–89.

18. Henri de Mondeville, "Chirurgie de Maître Henri de Mondeville,

composée de 1306 à 1320," in S. J. Reiser, A. J. Dyke, and W. J. Curran, eds., *Ethics in Medicine: Historical Perspectives and Contemporary Concerns* (Cambridge, Mass.: MIT Press, 1977), p. 15.

19. See A. R. Jonsen and S. E. Toulmin, *The Abuse of Casuistry* (Berkeley: University of California Press, 1988), p. 171; Jakobovits, *Jewish Medical Ethics,* pp. 49—52.

20. Marcia Angell, "Physicians and Cost Containment," *Journal of the American Medical Association* 254 (1985): 1203.

21. Aristotle, *Nicomachean Ethics* 5.1.1129a.

22. Giovanni Codronchus, *De Christiana ac Tuta Medendi Ratione* (1591), I, 43.

3. The Nobility of Medicine

1. Harvey Cushing, *The Life of Sir William Osler* (Oxford: Clarendon Press, 1925), II, 275.

2. Ibid., p. 281.

3. James Walsh, *The Thirteenth, Greatest of Centuries* (New York: Catholic Summer School Press, 1907).

4. Cushing, *Life of Osler,* p. 391.

5. William Osler, "Chauvinism in Medicine," *Montreal Medical Journal* 31 (1902): 684.

6. Charles Singer, *A Short History of Medicine* (Oxford: Oxford University Press, 1962), p. 626.

7. Chauncey Leake, ed., *Percival's Medical Ethics* (Huntington, N.Y.: Krieger, 1976), p. 71.

8. Robert B. Bean and William B. Bean, eds., *Sir William Osler's Aphorisms from His Bedside Teachings and Writings* (Springfield, Ill.: Charles C Thomas, 1968), p. 88.

9. Richard C. Cabot, "The Use of Truth and Falsehood in Medicine: An Experimental Study," *American Medicine* 5 (1903): 334—339.

10. Osler, "Chauvinism in Medicine," p. 684.

11. William Osler, "British Medicine in Greater Britain," *Montreal Medical Journal* 26 (1897): 186.

12. Bean and Bean, *Sir William Osler's Aphorisms,* p. 113.
13. Edgar Hume, *The Medical Work of the Knights Hospitallers of Saint John of Jerusalem* (Baltimore: Johns Hopkins Press, 1940). References to the Rule of the Knights can be found in this volume.
14. Jonathan Riley-Smith, *The Knights of Saint John in Jerusalem and Cyprus* (New York: Macmillan, 1976), p. 331.
15. Ludwig Edelstein, *Ancient Medicine* (Baltimore: Johns Hopkins Press, 1967), pp. 319–348.
16. Will Durant, *The Age of Faith* (New York: Simon and Schuster, 1950), pp. 555–558.
17. Code of Ethics of the American Medical Association (1847), chap. 1, art. 1, par. 1, in Leake, *Percival's Medical Ethics,* p. 219.
18. Bean and Bean, *Sir William Osler's Aphorisms,* p. 63.
19. "Doctors and Patients: Image vs. Reality," *Time,* July 31, 1989, pp. 48, 50.

4. Doctor Locke and Doctors' Rights

1. Robert Berenson, "Meet Dr. Squeezed," *New York Times,* July 21, 1989.
2. Robert Sade, "Medical Care as a Right: A Refutation," *New England Journal of Medicine* 285 (1971): 1288–92; quotation on p. 1289.
3. Kenneth Dewhurst, *John Locke, Physician and Philosopher* (London: Wellcome Historical Medical Library, 1963).
4. Henry Sigerest, *The Great Doctors* (New York: Dover Publications, 1933), p. 181.
5. Ernest Barker, *Social Contract* (New York: Oxford University Press, 1962), p. xvi.
6. John Locke, *Second Treatise on Civil Government,* ed. Peter Laslett (Cambridge, Mass.: Harvard University Press, 1966), secs. 27, 87, 149.
7. Norman Gevitz, ed., *Other Healers: Unorthodox Medicine in America* (Baltimore: Johns Hopkins University Press, 1988).

8. See Paul Starr, *The Social Transformation of American Medicine* (New York: Basic Books, 1982).

9. Principles of Medical Ethics of the American Medical Association (1903), chap. 3, sec. 1, in Chauncey Leake, ed., *Percival's Medical Ethics* (Huntington, N.Y.: Krieger, 1976), p. 241.

10. Ronald Numbers, "The Third Party: Health Insurance in America," in M. J. Vogel and Charles Rosenberg, eds., *The Therapeutic Revolution* (Philadelphia: University of Pennsylvania Press, 1979).

11. Locke, *Second Treatise*, sec. 27.

12. C. B. Macpherson, *The Political Theory of Possessive Individualism: Hobbes to Locke* (Oxford: Clarendon Press, 1962).

13. Richard Harris, *A Sacred Trust* (New York: New American Library, 1966).

14. Sade, "Medical Care as a Right," p. 1289.

5. Bentham in His Box

1. Jeremy Bentham, *Correspondence,* I, 136, quoted in Ross Harrison, *Bentham* (London: Routledge and Kegan Paul, 1983), p. 6.

2. *New York Times,* June 18, 1986.

3. William McNeill, *People and Plagues* (Garden City, N.Y.: Doubleday Anchor Books, 1976), p. 273.

4. See Michael Bayles, *Contemporary Utilitarianism* (Garden City, N.Y.: Doubleday Anchor Books, 1968).

5. Nicholas Rescher, "The Allocation of Exotic Life Saving Therapy," in S. J. Reiser, A. J. Dyke, and W. J. Curran, *Ethics in Medicine: Historical Perspectives and Contemporary Concerns* (Cambridge, Mass.: MIT Press, 1977), p. 616.

6. G. J. Warnock, *The Object of Morality* (London: Methuen, 1971), p. 33.

7. Peter Singer, *Practical Ethics* (Cambridge: Cambridge University Press, 1979), p. 134.

8. M. P. Mack, *Jeremy Bentham: An Odyssey of Ideas* (New York: Columbia University Press, 1963), p. 237.

9. Daniel Bell, "Toward the Year 2000: Work in Progress," *Daedalus* 96 (1967): 43.

10. Victor Ferkiss, *Technological Man* (New York: Braziller, 1969), pp. 37–38.

11. C. S. Singer and E. A. Underwood, *A Short History of Medicine* (Oxford: Oxford University Press, 1962), p. 722.

6. *The Snake and the Saints*

1. "Doctors and Patients: Image vs. Reality," *Time,* July 31, 1989, pp. 48–51.

2. Jan Schouten, *The Rod and Serpent of Asklepios* (Amsterdam: Elsevier, 1967), p. 2.

3. Charles Kerenyi, *Asklepios* (New York: Pantheon Books, 1958), p. 34.

4. Hippocrates, *Aphorisms* 1; *Precepts* 8.

5. Hippocrates, *Art* 1.

6. G. J. Warnock, *The Object of Morality* (London: Methuen, 1971), chap. 2; quotations on p. 26.

7. Kerenyi, *Asklepios,* pp. 26–27.

8. Hippocrates, *Decorum* 32.

9. J. H. Oliver and P. L. Maas, "An Ancient Poem on the Duties of a Physician," *Bulletin of the History of Medicine* 7 (1939): 315.

7. *Humanities Are the Hormones*

1. William Osler, *The Old Humanities and the New Science* (Boston: Houghton Mifflin, 1920), pp. 26, 28.

2. Ibid., pp. 25–26.

3. V. C. Medvei, *A History of Endocrinology* (Boston: MTP Press, 1982), p. 342.

4. T. E. Andreoli et al., *Cecil's Essentials of Medicine* (Philadelphia: W. B. Saunders, 1986), p. 1216.

5. Osler, *The Old Humanities,* pp. 36, 38.

6. Charles E. Odegaard, *Dear Doctor: A Personal Letter to a Physician* (Menlo Park, Calif.: Henry J. Kaiser Foundation, 1986), p. 38.

7. Eric Cassell, *The Place of Humanities in Medicine* (Hastings-on-Hudson, N.Y.: Hastings Center, 1984), p. 10.

8. Association of American Medical Colleges, *Physicians for the Twenty-First Century* (Washington, D.C.: AAMC, 1984), p. 5.

9. Edmund Pellegrino, *Humanism and the Physician* (Knoxville: University of Tennessee Press, 1979); Cassell, *The Place of Humanities;* Odegaard, *Dear Doctor.*

10. R. L. Memmler and D. L. Wood, *The Human Body in Health and Disease* (Philadelphia: Lippincott, 1983), p. 295.

11. Andreoli et al., *Cecil's Essentials,* p. 460.

12. Odegaard, *Dear Doctor,* p. 45.

13. President's Commission for the Study of Ethical Problems in Medicine and in Biomedical and Behavioral Research, *Deciding to Forego Life-Sustaining Treatment* (Washington, D.C.: Government Printing Office, 1983), pp. 82–89.

14. William Pfaff, "Reflections," *New Yorker,* December 7, 1987, p. 150.

Index

Index